£1

Past Papers

MRCOG Part Two Multiple Choice Questions, 1997–2001

Royal College of Obstetricians and Gynaecologists Examination Committee

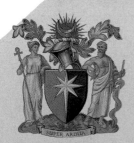

RCOG Press
May 2004

i

Published by the **RCOG Press** at the Royal College of Obstetricians and Gynaecologists, 27 Sussex Place, Regent's Park, London NW1 4RG

www.rcog.org.uk

Registered charity no. 213280

First published 2004

ISBN 1-904752-03-9

RCOG Press Editor: Wasseema Malik

Design: FiSH Books
Printed by Latimer Trend & Co Ltd. Estover Road, Plymouth PL6 7PL

Introduction

As a contribution to self-directed learning for the Multiple Choice Question papers in the Part 1 and Part 2 MRCOG examinations, the Royal College of Obstetricians and Gynaecologists has decided to publish ten past papers. Answers are not included because we would like to encourage candidates to seek out information themselves and thus learn in the process.

For Part 2 MRCOG, pilot or 'test' questions are not included in the final mark and have therefore been excluded from these papers and the remaining questions renumbered sequentially. The papers are otherwise published as they appeared in the examination. Subsequent editorial or content changes may have been undertaken before any questions were reused in the examination. No responsibility may be taken for the content or terminology of the questions, as phraseology may change over time.

There is no negative marking in the examination, so all questions should be attempted. Failure to respond to every question may result in inadvertent loss of marks.

The content of this book remains copyright of the Royal College of Obstetricians and Gynaecologists.

Examination Committee
April 2004

Contents

March 1997   1

September 1997   16

March 1998   32

September 1998   47

March 1999   65

September 1999   84

March 2000   103

September 2000   120

March 2001   135

September 2001   153

Contents

March 197
September 199 ... 19
March 199 ... 32
... 47
March 199 ... 63
September 199 ... 84
... 105
November 200 ... 120
March 200 ... 135
... 151

March 1997

Achondroplasia

1. is the most common lethal chondrodysplasia.
2. can be excluded by a normal fetal femur length measured by ultrasound at 18 weeks of pregnancy.
3. is associated with polyhydramnios.
4. is not associated with mental retardation.

Phenytoin

5. is best administered by intramuscular injection.
6. has a short biological half-life.
7. is rapidly absorbed from the intestinal tract.
8. is metabolised by the liver.

Neonatal jaundice appearing on the third day and still present at two weeks of age may be due to

9. haemolytic disease of the newborn due to rhesus incompatibility.
10. galactosaemia.
11. phenylketonuria.
12. neonatal hyperthyroidism.

Analysis of a sample of amniotic fluid obtained by amniocentesis assists in the diagnosis of

13. Tay-Sachs disease.
14. congenital adrenal hyperplasia.
15. spina bifida occulta.
16. oesophageal atresia.

The following diseases are inherited as autosomal recessive traits:

17. pseudohypertrophic (Duchenne) muscular dystrophy.
18. cystic fibrosis.
19. haemophilia.

20.   phenylketonuria.
21.   congenital spherocytosis.

Factors predisposing to maternal pulmonary aspiration of gastric contents during labour include

22.   an increase in gastric motility.
23.   the effect of progesterone on the cardiac sphincter.
24.   epidural analgesia.
25.   the use of muscle relaxant

Intrahepatic cholestasis in pregnancy is characteristically associated with

26.   elevated serum concentrations of the direct bilirubin fraction.
27.   a positive direct Coombs test in the neonate.
28.   elevated serum acid phosphatase activity.

The following statements concerning preterm labour are correct:

29.   Maternal administration of steroids is contraindicated in cases with prolonged rupture of membranes.
30.   Women with a history of subfertility have an increased risk.
31.   Babies weighing between 500–1000 g should be delivered by caesarean section.

Severe pregnancy-induced hypertension is characteristically associated with

32.   a reduced uric acid clearance.
33.   abnormally high maternal concentrations of serum cortisol.
34.   hypernatraemia.

Complications arising during the administration of ritodrine are more likely when there is

35.   maternal anaemia of less than 9 g/dl.
36.   rupture of the membranes.
37.   maternal diabetes.

Rubella infection in the first trimester of pregnancy is associated with a subsequent increased risk of

38.   phocomelia.
39.   intrauterine growth retardation.

40.   oligohydramnios.
41.   neonatal purpura.

In a prospective blind study of a possible new method of antenatal screening for a particular fetal disorder, 60,000 consecutive pregnant women were recruited and tested. One hundred of the fetuses were found to be affected. The test had a sensitivity of 90% and a specificity of 95%. Based on this study the following statements are correct:

42.   A woman with a positive test has a 10% chance of having an affected child.
43.   The results demonstrate that the test fulfils the criteria set by the World Health Organization for screening.
44.   95% of affected cases had a positive screening test.
45.   The negative predictive rate can be calculated from the data provided.
46.   The false positive rate can be calculated using Fisher's exact test.

Nuchal translucency

47.   is more obvious at eight weeks than at 11 weeks of gestation.
48.   is diagnostic of a chromosomal abnormality.
49.   is a marker for a neural tube defect.

Cerebral palsy may only be attributed to intrapartum events if

50.   the neonate exhibits signs of moderate or severe ischaemic encephalopathy with hypoxic injury to other organs.
51.   the neurological condition can only be explained by intrapartum events.
52.   there is evidence of prolonged intrapartum asphyxia.
53.   other causes have been excluded by computed tomography or magnetic resonance imaging.

With regard to fetal growth and birth weight,

54.   a high carbohydrate intake in early pregnancy suppresses placental growth.
55.   a high intake of iron and folate supplements in late pregnancy is associated with higher birth weight.
56.   there is a significant association between fetal and placental weight.

The following are recognised to be of proven benefit:

57. appropriate antibiotic treatment during labour to women with current beta-haemolytic streptococcal colonisation of the vagina.
58. administration of anti-D immunoglobulin to rhesus-negative women at 28 and 34 weeks of gestation.
59. external cephalic version after 36 completed weeks of pregnancy.
60. immunotherapy with paternal leucocytes to prevent recurrent miscarriage.
61. elective forceps delivery for preterm birth.

Features of disseminated intravascular coagulation include

62. activation of factor VII.
63. the appearance of free plasmin in the circulation.
64. reversal of the process by transfusion of stored whole blood.

In a pregnant woman over the age of 35 years, there is a recognised increase in the

65. incidence of pregnancy prolonged beyond 40 weeks of gestation.
66. frequency of multiple pregnancy.
67. incidence of maternal hyperthyroidism.

Jaundice is a recognised feature of the following conditions of the newborn:

68. sickle cell disease.
69. beta-thalassaemia.
70. cytomegalovirus infection.
71. congenital spherocytosis.

Features of sickle cell haemoglobin C disease in pregnancy include

72. a characteristic association with anaemia.
73. splenomegaly.
74. fat embolus.
75. infarction of bone.

Congenital rubella syndrome in the neonate

76. is likely to follow accidental vaccination of the mother with rubella vaccine in the first trimester.
77. commonly includes patent ductus arteriosus.
78. may result in excretion of the rubella virus for more than six months.

79. includes intracranial calcification.
80. includes neonatal purpura.

The following statements relating to toxoplasmosis and pregnancy are correct:

81. Severe disease in the fetus is most likely to occur if the mother acquires the infection during the first two trimesters of pregnancy.
82. Among mothers known to have acquired toxoplasmosis during the first trimester of pregnancy the spontaneous abortion rate is above 20%.
83. If antibodies are present before conception, the fetus will be unaffected.

Intravenous ergometrine when given as a bolus for the third stage of labour is characteristically associated with

84. a fall in mean arterial blood pressure.
85. a rise in peripheral resistance.
86. vomiting.

The following conditions are characteristically associated with a reduction in uteroplacental blood flow:

87. maternal respiratory alkalosis.
88. the second stage of labour.
89. maternal pulmonary hypertension.
90. cord presentation.

Eye damage is a recognised consequence of fetal infection with

91. *Treponema pallidum.*
92. *Toxoplasma gondii.*
93. the Epstein-Barr virus.

With a breech presentation,

94. the risk of significant congenital anomaly at 30 weeks of gestation is less than 5%.
95. the incidence is greater with delivery at the 30th week than at 38 weeks of gestation.
96. congenital hip dislocation is unrelated to route of delivery.
97. a boy is more at risk of congenital hip dislocation than is a girl.

An increased risk of fetal malformation is associated with

98. poliomyelitis vaccine administered in early pregnancy.
99. diagnostic amniocentesis.
100. warfarin sodium administration.
101. smoking 20 cigarettes or more a day.
102. rubella vaccination in the first trimester of pregnancy.

A previously normotensive primigravida has developed a blood pressure of 150/100 mmHg and 4 g of proteinuria per 24 hours. The following findings would be consistent with the above:

103. loss of diurnal variation in blood pressure.
104. a creatinine clearance of 120–150 ml/minute.
105. hyperreflexia.
106. a raised concentration of fibrin degradation products (FDP).
107. epigastric pain.

In the management of the infant with suspected rhesus haemolytic disease,

108. a positive maternal Kleihauer test indicates the need for exchange transfusion.
109. the mature infant is more susceptible than the premature to kernicterus.

The secretion of breast milk is decreased by the administration of

110. metoclopramide.
111. warfarin sodium.
112. methadone.
113. depot medroxyprogesterone acetate.

Acute inversion of the uterus

114. is a recognised complication of ergometrine administration.
115. is a recognised consequence of genital prolapse.

The following conditions would be expected to conform to the pattern of inheritance shown in Figure 1:

116. achondroplasia.
117. phenylketonuria.
118. neurofibromatosis.
119. cystic fibrosis.
120. myotonic dystrophy.

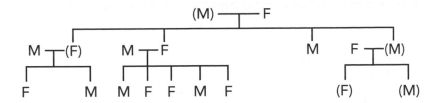

[M = normal male, (M) = affected male, F = normal female, (F) = affected female]

Figure 1

In the diagnosis and management of amniotic fluid infection following rupture of the membranes before the onset of labour

121. the most common causative organism is the group A haemolytic streptococcus.
122. 24 hours of antibiotic therapy is advisable prior to delivery.
123. the absence of maternal pyrexia precludes the diagnosis.
124. oxytocin is contraindicated to induce labour.

Necrotising enterocolitis is characterised by

125. blood in the stool.
126. abdominal distension.
127. bile-stained vomit.
128. an association with preterm birth.
129. an association with severe intrauterine growth retardation.

The following lesion is correctly paired with a recognised clinical association:

130. A maternal serum alphafetoprotein concentration : gastroschisis of more than three times the median.

A primigravid patient is delivered by lower-segment caesarean section for fetal distress. In a second pregnancy,

131. the risk of rupture of the uterine scar in labour is approximately 5%.
132. epidural analgesia during labour is contraindicated.

A healthy normotensive woman aged 40 years is pregnant for the first time. Compared with an otherwise similar 25-year-old woman

133. it is significantly more likely that she will have a higher fasting blood glucose concentration.
134. she has an increased chance of developing a trophoblastic tumour.
135. the risk of ectopic pregnancy is increased three-fold.
136. the risk of her baby having a neural tube defect is increased by 10%.

Perinatal mortality in the United Kingdom

137. is defined as all stillbirths and all deaths in the first 28 days after birth.
138. is associated with low-birthweight (less than 2.5 kg) babies in over 60% of cases.
139. is lower in babies of mothers who are primiparous.

The following maternal infections may be transmitted to the newborn as a result of vaginal delivery:

140. human immunodeficiency virus.
141. human papillomavirus.
142. *Listeria monocytogenes.*
143. malaria.

The following statements regarding toxoplasmosis are correct:

144. A positive specific anti-toxoplasma immunoglobulin M test in the serum of the pregnant woman indicates an acute infection.
145. The incidence of toxoplasma infections in pregnant women in the UK is about 2/1000 pregnancies.
146. About 95% of maternal toxoplasma infections are transmitted to the fetus.
147. Spiramycin is used in the treatment of *in utero* toxoplasma infections.
148. Toxoplasma gondii is a cause of repeated abortions.

The following conditions are correctly paired with an appropriate treatment:

149. Primary ovarian failure : clomifene citrate.
150. Puerperal mastitis : danazol.
151. Secondary ovarian failure : human chorionic gonadotrophin.
152. Precocious puberty : luteinising hormone releasing hormone analogue.

The following symptoms are correctly paired with a recognised cause:

153. Anosmia : polycystic ovarian disease.
154. Diplopia : avascular necrosis of the pituitary.

In primary carcinoma of the fallopian tube,

155. the tumour is bilateral in approximately 60% of cases.
156. the largest number of reported cases occur in the sixth decade of life.
157. transcoelomic spread rarely occurs.
158. radiotherapy is the treatment of choice.
159. a profuse watery vaginal discharge is a characteristic symptom.

Isolated gonadotrophin deficiency (Kallman syndrome)

160. is due to failure of development of the gonadotrophin cells of the pituitary.
161. is a recognised cause of secondary amenorrhoea.
162. is characteristically associated with nerve deafness.

With regard to weight-related amenorrhoea,

163. prepubertal self-imposed weight loss cannot delay puberty.
164. gonadotrophin secretion is above normal at the time of gross weight loss.
165. clomifene citrate stimulation tests are usually negative.

Following vasectomy,

166. plasma testosterone concentration shows a significant decline in the first six months.
167. there is a positive correlation with subsequent gall bladder disease.
168. the failure rate is approximately 2/1000.
169. sperm autoantibodies develop in at least 40% of patients.
170. epididymo-orchitis is the most common immediate side effect.

Anovulation is characteristically associated with

171. dysmenorrhoea.
172. endometriosis.
173. premenstrual tension.
174. chronic renal failure.

Recognised causes of postmenopausal bleeding include

175. preinvasive carcinoma of the cervix.
176. benign teratoma of the ovary.
177. atrophic vaginitis.
178. hepatic cirrhosis.
179. phaeochromocytoma.

Recognised complications of the intrauterine contraceptive devices include

180. spontaneous expulsion in 30% during the first three months following insertion.
181. an increased incidence of endometriosis.

The following statements concerning intestinal obstruction are correct:

182. Gas demonstrated radiologically throughout the small and large bowel is a feature of paralytic ileus.
183. Obstruction due to Crohn's disease is not commonly associated with pain.

There is an increased risk of endometrial carcinoma in a patient who has

184. a past history of habitual abortion.
185. a granulosa-cell tumour of the ovary.
186. an early menopause.
187. never had a cervical smear.
188. had immunosuppressive therapy.

Recognised complications of gynaecological laparoscopy include

189. puncture of common iliac blood vessels.
190. surgical emphysema.
191. haemoperitoneum.
192. damage to the anterior division of the lumbosacral plexus.
193. puncture of the inferior epigastric artery.

A 30-year-old woman, who had been taking the combined oral contraceptive pill for four years, stopped it one year ago, as she wished to become pregnant. Since then, her periods have occurred every 9–12 weeks. On examination, she is thin and anxious. She measures 1.52 m in height and weighs 41.5 kg, giving her a body mass index of 18 (normal range 19–26). On examination, the abdomen and pelvis are normal. Her partner has a normal semen analysis. In relation to this patient, the following statements are correct:

194. The delay in conception is likely to be significantly related to her long-term use of the contraceptive pill.
195. Significant weight gain is likely to restore a regular menstrual cycle.
196. Human menopausal gonadotrophin therapy is the treatment of choice.
197. Ovarian biopsy should be carried out at the time of laparoscopy.

In stage IIb carcinoma of the cervix,

198. the peak incidence is at 55–65 years of age.
199. radiotherapy is the treatment of choice.
200. less than 20% of patients will have lymph node involvement.
201. lymphangiography is helpful in the clinical staging.

In the androgen insensitivity syndrome (testicular feminisation),

202. infrequent scanty menstrual bleeding may occur.
203. body hair distribution is of the male type.
204. a familial incidence is recognised.

Recognised features of Turner syndrome include

205. coarctation of the aorta.
206. elevated serum gonadotrophin concentration.
207. a normal female karyotype.
208. red–green colour blindness.

The level of serum prolactin is

209. increased by exogenous thyrotrophin-releasing hormone.
210. increased in acromegaly.
211. depressed by levodopa administration.
212. increased by the administration of ergometrine.

Characteristics of atypical endometrial hyperplasia include

213. secretory changes in the endometrium.
214. ovulatory cycles.
215. hirsutism.
216. premenstrual tension.
217. an association with uterine fibroids.

Untreated female genital tuberculosis is characteristically associated with

218. recurrent abortion.
219. a primary source of infection in the lung.

The serum luteinising hormone (LH) concentration is raised in

220. anorexia nervosa.
221. polycystic ovarian disease.
222. cystadenocarcinoma of the ovary.
223. ovarian agenesis.
224. acromegaly.

The symptom of urge incontinence in women

225. is associated with a low intravesical pressure.
226. is associated with congenital shortening of the urethra.

Dysgerminomas of the ovary characteristically

227. have a peak prevalence in women under 30 years of age.
228. exhibit lymphoid infiltration of the fibrous stroma.
229. are radiosensitive.
230. are bilateral.
231. have a recognised association with hirsutism.

Cancer of the endometrium characteristically metastasises to the

232. brain.
233. para-aortic lymph nodes.
234. pouch of Douglas.
235. lungs.
236. liver.

The following statements about methods of contraception are correct:

237. The arcing diaphragm is the most suitable diaphragm to use in the presence of malpositions of the uterus.
238. Most diaphragms are impregnated with nonoxynol-9.
239. The male condom has a higher failure rate when used by uncircumcised men.
240. Cervical caps are associated with an increase of cervical ectopy.

Primary amenorrhoea is a characteristic feature of

241. congenital adrenal hyperplasia.
242. triple X karyotype.
243. Down syndrome.

Septic abortion, when associated with a *Clostridium perfringens* (*welchii*) infection, has the following recognised features:

244. disseminated intravascular coagulation.
245. acute renal failure.
246. haemolysis.
247. hyperpyrexia.
248. acute respiratory distress syndrome.

Recognised associations of secondary amenorrhoea include

249. prolonged administration of progestogens.
250. hyperthyroidism.
251. active pulmonary tuberculosis.
252. anorexia nervosa.
253. intrauterine synaechiae (Asherman syndrome).

Characteristic features of adenocarcinoma of the endocervix include

254. pyometra.
255. radiosensitivity.
256. a favourable response to methotrexate.
257. a positive Schiller's test.

Painless haematuria is a characteristic feature of

258. transitional-cell carcinoma of the bladder.
259. acute glomerulonephritis.
260. *Schistosoma haematobium* infection.

Recognised associations exist between pruritus ani and

261. diverticulitis coli.
262. Ascaris lumbricoides infestation.

Azoospermia associated with high concentrations of serum follicle-stimulating hormone (FSH) are characteristically found in the presence of

263. congenital absence of the vas deferens.
264. bilateral varicocele.
265. seminoma of the testis.

The following are recognised predisposing factors for secondary dysmenorrhoea:

266. endometrial resection.
267. congenital uterine anomalies.
268. fibroid polyps.
269. the presence of an intrauterine contraceptive device.

Clomifene citrate is a recognised treatment for

270. luteal phase deficiency.
271. oligozoospermia associated with a raised serum FSH concentration.
272. the resistant ovary syndrome

Osteoporosis

273. is associated with normal mineralisation of bone.
274. is likely to occur following a premature menopause.
275. is typically associated with bone deformity as opposed to fracture.
276. is a recognised feature of Cushing's syndrome.
277. is more common in smokers than in non-smokers.

Dual-channel cystometry

278. can distinguish neuropathic from idiopathic detrusor instability.
279. is dependent upon the measurement of urethral and intravesical pressures.

The climacteric

280. is associated with a sudden reduction in the concentration of plasma oestradiol.
281. is preceded by the cessation of the production of luteinising hormone.

Following the evacuation of a non-invasive (complete) hydatidiform mole,

282. combined oral contraceptive therapy has been reported to increase the need for chemotherapy.
283. a subsequent normal pregnancy obviates the need for further human chorionic gonadotrophin (hCG) assay.
284. there is a risk of choriocarcinoma developing in more than 20% of cases.
285. the use of an intrauterine contraceptive device is contraindicated.

Characteristic features of idiopathic female hirsutism include

286. elevated concentrations of serum FSH.
287. total serum testosterone concentrations above 4 nmol/l (normal range 1–2.8 nmol/l).
288. galactorrhoea.
289. oligomenorrhoea.

Cervical ectopy (erosion)

290. is more common in progestogen-only oral contraceptive users than in users of intrauterine contraceptive devices.

Condylomata accuminata

291. are most commonly found at the fourchette.
292. tend to regress during pregnancy.

Concerning 'genuine stress incontinence' and its treatment:

293. It can objectively be cured by a Burch-type colposuspension in more than 80% of cases (with no previous surgical treatment).
294. There is a 10% chance of detrusor instability developing in the year following a suspension procedure.
295. It can objectively be cured by an anterior vaginal repair in more than 80% of cases (with no previous surgical treatment).
296. Persistent voiding difficulty occurs in less than 5% of cases after suspension procedures.

Vaginal ultrasound will routinely detect

297. submucous fibroids of greater than 5-mm diameter.
298. a bicornuate uterus.
299. early endometrial carcinoma in a postmenopausal woman.
300. endometriosis in the pouch of Douglas.

September 1997

The following are typically inherited as an X-linked trait:

1. achondroplasia.
2. Huntington's chorea.
3. glucose-6-phosphate dehydrogenase deficiency.
4. von Willebrand's disease.
5. phenylketonuria.

The following statements regarding thyrotoxicosis complicating pregnancy and the puerperium are correct:

6. Drug therapy can be reliably monitored by the sole use of serial estimations of total serum thyroxine concentration.
7. Anti-thyroid drugs should be replaced by propranolol in the last four weeks of pregnancy.
8. Neonatal thyrotoxicosis is clinically apparent within 24 hours of birth.
9. Breastfeeding is contraindicated if a mother is taking propylthiouracil.
10. When mild, it cannot be distinguished clinically from normal pregnancy.

The following statements relating to vaccination are correct:

11. Human varicella zoster immunoglobulin should be given to the term newborn of a mother who has had shingles during the second trimester.
12. If vaccination against poliomyelitis is required in pregnancy, the Sabin strain should be employed.
13. Human varicella zoster immunoglobulin should be given to the term newborn of a mother who has had chickenpox during the second trimester.
14. Rabies vaccine is safe for use in pregnancy.
15. Tetanus vaccination carries no risk of intrauterine fetal infection.

Concerning toxoplasmosis,

16. it is transmitted from mother to fetus in less than 10% of cases.
17. it is transmitted by ingestion of raw, poorly washed vegetables.
18. it is treatable during pregnancy.

Listeria infection in the pregnant woman is characteristically associated with

19. severe diarrhoea.
20. meconium staining of the amniotic fluid.
21. sensitivity to amoxicillin.

Characteristic features of megaloblastic anaemia of pregnancy include

22. a more rapid fall in haemoglobin level than in microcytic anaemia.
23. a risk of subacute combined degeneration of the spinal cord in untreated cases.
24. a prompt response to hydroxycobalamin.
25. an associated histamine fast achlorhydria.
26. the presence of circulating antibodies to gastric parietal cells.

Concerning anaemia in pregnancy (excluding the haemoglobinopathies),

27. red-cell folate estimation provides more useful information than does the plasma folate concentration.
28. serum ferritin concentration is raised in iron-deficiency anaemia.
29. a microcytic blood film excludes folate deficiency.

The following statements regarding epilepsy complicating pregnancy are correct:

30. Estimation of salivary anticonvulsant concentrations is more reliable than estimation of blood concentrations in monitoring drug dosage.
31. Epidural analgesia is contraindicated.

In patients undergoing anticoagulation with warfarin sodium,

32. the effects of the drug are antagonised within ten minutes by intravenous administration of vitamin K.
33. breastfeeding is contraindicated.

A rhesus-negative woman is in the 31st week of her fourth pregnancy. Her third baby was stillborn at 38 weeks due to haemolytic disease. Her husband's genotype is CDE/cde. In her current pregnancy

34. a decision to perform an intrauterine transfusion will be based upon the serum antibody titre.
35. she requires 250 iu anti-D immunoglobulin within 48 hours of delivery.
36. there is a 50% chance that her baby will be rhesus negative.

Recognised associations of major pulmonary thromboembolism include

37. protein C deficiency.
38. early change in the chest X-ray.
39. an inverted T wave on electrocardiogram.

Recognised features of sickle cell disease complicating pregnancy include

40. an increased incidence of iron deficiency.
41. fat embolism.

Translocation Down syndrome is characterised by

42. coarctation of the aorta.
43. a greater paternal genetic component than trisomy 21.
44. maternal age over 35 years.

Congenital dislocation of the hip is characteristically

45. more common in girls than boys.
46. bilateral in more than 50% of cases.
47. associated with persistent breech presentation.

Recognised associations of persistent ductus arteriosus in the neonate include

48. the administration of indomethacin prenatally.
49. Marfan syndrome.

Neonatal jaundice appearing 12 hours after delivery is a recognised feature of

50. atresia of the bile ducts.
51. urinary tract infection.

In the preterm baby

52. with haemolytic disease, exchange transfusion should be considered at serum bilirubin concentrations lower than those for term babies.
53. pneumothorax is a recognised sequel to pulmonary interstitial emphysema.
54. the commonest intracranial complication is subarachnoid haemorrhage.
55. planned forceps delivery is advised to facilitate any vaginal delivery.

Hydrops fetalis (not due to rhesus isoimmunisation) is a recognised complication of

56. parvovirus infection.
57. cystic adenomatoid malformation of the lung.
58. fetal paroxysmal tachycardia.

Concerning hyperemesis,

59. the severity of the condition relates directly to serum levels of human chorionic gonadotrophin.
60. it can lead to the development of Wernicke's encephalopathy.
61. it is associated with transient hypothyroidism in about 5% of cases.

Abdominal cervical cerclage

62. should be removed at approximately 36 weeks of gestation.
63. should not be carried out prior to 16 weeks of gestation.

Chorionic villus sampling (CVS)

64. facilitates prenatal diagnosis of spina bifida.
65. is optimally performed before eight weeks of gestation.
66. is associated with a higher false positive rate than is amniocentesis.

Diagnostic amniocentesis at 16 weeks of gestation is associated with an increased incidence of

67. hare lip and cleft palate.

68. neonatal respiratory difficulty.
69. meconium ileus.

Chorioamnionitis

70. is characteristically associated with anaerobic organisms.
71. does not occur in the presence of intact membranes.

Recognised causes of polyhydramnios include

72. polycystic disease of the fetal kidney.
73. *Listeria monocytogenes* infection.
74. diaphragmatic hernia.

In the management of massive haemorrhage in the labour ward,

75. if additional calcium is needed, then 10% calcium chloride should be given.
76. colloid solutions are preferable to crystalloid solutions to expand plasma volume.
77. platelet concentrates should be transfused at an early stage.
78. fresh frozen plasma should be given at an early stage.

Abnormally high serum concentrations of human chorionic gonadotrophin (hCG) in pregnancy are associated with

79. fetal erythroblastosis.
80. carneous mole.

Monozygotic twinning is

82. a recognised cause of acute polyhydramnios occurring in the second trimester.
83. familial.
84. associated with a common amniotic sac in about 25% of cases.
85. always monochorionic.

An increased intake of folic acid is required when pregnancy is associated with

86. intrauterine growth retardation.
87. the administration of ampicillin.
88. sickle cell disease.
89. malaria.
90. maternal coeliac disease.

In the pregnant woman of 35 years or over there is an increased incidence of

91.   anencephaly.
92.   breech presentation.
93.   fatal thromboembolism.
94.   dizygotic twins.
95.   acute appendicitis.

Contraindications to the use of epidural analgesia include

96.   hypertension treated with labetalol.
97.   a previous history of deep vein thrombosis.
98.   maternal mitral stenosis.

With regard to oblique lie of the fetus,

99.   at term, dorso-anterior are more frequent than dorso-posterior positions.
100.   there is a recognised association with fetal renal agenesis.
101.   arm prolapse occurs more frequently than cord prolapse.
102.   stabilising induction before term is indicated.

Forty pregnant patients participated in a randomised controlled trial of complete bed rest versus ambulation in the management of proteinuric hypertension. The measurement of urinary oestriol (nmol/litre) in the two groups was as follows:

	Rested group (n = 20)	Ambulant group (n = 20)
Mean	209.9	365.6
Standard deviation	70.3	197.1
Range	180–1200	115–860

$t = 2.08$; difference between 'means' = 155.7; $P = 0.022$

The following statements, which refer to the above data, are correct:

103.   In the study described, patients were allocated alternately to 'rested' and 'ambulant' groups.
104.   The value of '$P = 0.022$' suggests that the observed difference did not occur by chance.
105.   The value of 't' refers to a test for the difference between the means.

106. Among the 'ambulant' group, 95% of oestriol values were between 365.6 ± 197.1.
107. The standard error of the mean for the 'rested' group was 280.2.

Intramuscular pethidine in labour

108. is eliminated from the neonate within 24 hours of delivery.
109. produces maximal neonatal respiratory depression if given within the hour before delivery.
110. slows maternal gastric emptying.

The following statements regarding the maternal cardiovascular system in pregnancy are correct:

111. In patients with uncorrected chronic rheumatic valvular heart disease, crystalline penicillin given alone provides adequate antibiotic prophylaxis.
112. Supraventricular arrhythmias occur more often in the pregnant than in the nonpregnant woman.
113. Most murmurs first detected in pregnancy are due to mitral regurgitation.

Symptomatic intrahepatic cholestasis of pregnancy characteristically

114. occurs in the last trimester.
115. is associated with neonatal jaundice.
116. leads to pruritus in the absence of jaundice.
117. is associated with premature delivery.
118. is unlikely to recur in a subsequent pregnancy.

Placental abruption

119. occurs in approximately 10% of otherwise uncomplicated pregnancies.
120. occurs with increased frequency in women who smoke.
121. is directly related to folic acid deficiency.
122. is associated with antecedent hypertension in about 80% of cases.

The following statements concerning eclampsia are correct:

123. Antepartum eclampsia has a higher maternal mortality rate than has intrapartum eclampsia.
124. The fit occurs following delivery in less than 10% of cases.
125. If maternal death follows, the commonest cause is renal failure.

Ritodrine

126. has an effective dose range of 150–350 microgrammes/minute.
127. causes peripheral vasodilatation at therapeutic doses.
129. is less effective if used in the presence of ruptured membranes.
130. should be administered in a 5% dextrose solution.

The 47XXX karyotype

131. is a recognised cause of premature menopause.
132. has a recognised association with endometrial carcinoma.

Asymptomatic vaginal adenosis

133. has a diploid chromosomal pattern.
134. occurs only in patients with prenatal exposure to diethylstilboestrol.
135. is a recognised complication of herpes simplex virus type II infection.

Concerning continuous combined hormone replacement therapy (HRT):

136. It protects against endometrial cancer in postmenopausal women.
137. It is associated with breakthrough bleeding in less than 10% of women.
138. Women who develop breast cancer and have taken HRT are more likely to be alive ten years later than women who have never taken HRT.
139. It can only be prescribed by the oral route.

Concerning carcinoma of the vagina:

140. The commonest site for a primary tumour is in the upper third of the vagina.
141. Clear-cell adenocarcinomas are the commonest primary tumour.
142. The majority are metastatic.
143. Radiotherapy is the treatment of choice.

Cervical intraepithelial neoplasia stage 3 (CIN3) is characterised by

144. more rapid progression to invasive cancer during pregnancy.
145. loss of stratification and polarity in the epithelium.

Concerning pelvic irradiation for carcinoma of the cervix,

146. urinary tract injuries are more common than bowel injuries.
147. small bowel is more sensitive than large bowel.
148. the tolerance of normal tissues is enhanced by giving hyperbaric oxygen.
149. adenocarcinomas are more sensitive than squamous-cell carcinomas.
150. the prognosis is adversely affected by the presence of salpingitis.

Factors which are considered to predispose to the development of carcinoma of the endometrium include

151. previous radiation-induced menopause.
152. adrenal hyperplasia.

Choriocarcinoma

153. can be diagnosed with ultrasound.
154. can occur in the absence of a previous pregnancy.
155. even with optimal treatment, has a five-year survival rate of less than 70%.

Concentrations of serum CA125

156. are usually elevated in patients with ascites due to alcoholic cirrhosis.
157. are usually elevated in women with ovarian germ-cell tumours.
158. often rise transiently following an abdominal operation.
159. are a sign of poor prognosis if still elevated after chemotherapy.
160. frequently rise prior to clinical signs of relapse from ovarian cancer.

The diagnosis of borderline epithelial tumours of the ovary is made by

161. clinical examination.
162. measurement of tumour marker in the patient's serum.
163. computed tomography (CT scan).

In the treatment of ovarian cancer

164. infracolic omentectomy should be performed in stage II disease.
165. second-line chemotherapy often produces dramatic remission of the disease.
166. bowel resection is not justifiable.

The following statements concerning female cancers in the UK are correct:

167. The proportion of women with cancer of the ovary who will die from the condition is approximately 60%.
168. The proportion of women with cancer of the endometrium who will die from the disease is approximately 40%.
169. The lifetime risk of a woman developing breast cancer is approximately 10%.
170. The lifetime risk of a woman developing ovarian cancer is approximately 0.2%.

Recognised causes of vaginal bleeding in a girl aged seven years include

171. *trichomonas vaginitis.*
172. polyostotic fibrous dysplasia (Albright's syndrome).
173. craniopharyngioma.
174. postencephalitic syndrome.

Recognised associations of short stature in adolescent girls include

175. androgen insensitivity syndrome.
176. XXX karyotype.

In a 25-year-old woman, serum follicle-stimulating hormone concentration is characteristically raised in

177. acromegaly.
178. anorexia nervosa.
179. polycystic ovarian syndrome.
180. the presence of a granulosa cell tumour.

Hyperprolactinaemia is a recognised consequence of the administration of

181. chlorpromazine.
182. phenytoin.
183. amitriptyline.
184. metoclopramide.
185. alpha-methyldopa.

In a patient with a pituitary prolactinoma

187. impotence is a recognised feature in the male.
188. the tumour regresses during pregnancy.

Concerning delayed female puberty:

189. the treatment of choice is a 20-microgramme-containing combined oral contraceptive pill.
190. gonadotrophin-releasing hormone (GnRH) agonists can be administered in a pulsatile manner to induce development.
191. it is considered delayed if there is no pubic or axillary hair development by the age of 13 years.
192. it is associated with thalassaemia major.
193. it may be associated with a prolactinoma.

The following statements concerning vulval lichen sclerosus are correct:

194. Squamous-cell carcinoma of the vulva occurs in less than 10% of women with this disease.
195. It does not occur before puberty.
196. The use of a potent corticosteroid ointment is contraindicated with this disease.
197. A simple vulvectomy is appropriate management in uncomplicated cases.
198. It exclusively affects the vulva.

The following conditions affecting the gastrointestinal tract may also affect the vulva:

199. Crohn's disease.
200. ulcerative colitis.
201. diverticular disease.

Recognised causes of granulomatous lesions of the vulva include

202. Paget's disease.
203. lichen sclerosus.
204. Behçet's syndrome.

When a ureterovaginal fistula occurs after pelvic surgery

205. the serum urea concentration is elevated.
206. a characteristic feature is the presence of free fluid in the abdomen.

If ureteric transection is recognised at the time of pelvic surgery,

207. reimplantation directly into the bladder is most appropriate when transection has occurred at the level of the cervix.

208. the affected ureter should be ligated when the presence of the contralateral kidney has been confirmed.

When compared with radiotherapy, radical hysterectomy

209. is less favoured in patients with stage Ia carcinoma of the cervix.
210. carries a reduced risk of subsequent lymphocyst formation.
211. is preferable in younger patients with stage IIb carcinoma of the cervix.

The following statements concerning wound healing and suture materials are correct:

212. Chromic catgut retains some tensile strength for up to 30 days after the operation.
213. All absorbable suture materials are absorbed by hydrolysis.
214. In normal healing, skin regains 80% of its tensile strength by seven days.

Bacterial vaginosis

215. can be diagnosed on culture of a high vaginal swab.
216. is associated with an increased number of vaginal lactobacilli.
217. is associated with a vaginal pH above 5.
218. is associated with an increased number of anaerobes.
219. can be successfully treated with intravaginal clindamycin.

The following statements concerning the human immunodeficiency virus (HIV-I) are correct:

220. Sexual transmission is reduced by the use of spermicides.
221. It has a rate of transmission to the fetus in a seropositive mother of over 60%.

In a patient with chlamydial infection

222. lymphogranuloma venereum is a recognised clinical presentation.
223. neonatal conjunctivitis appears in the first 48 hours after birth.

Pelvic abscess is a recognised complication of

224. pyometra.
225. ulcerative colitis.

Late sequelae of salpingitis characteristically include

226. psoas abscess.
227. pyometra.

The risk of fatal postoperative thromboembolism is

228. increased in patients with blood group O compared with those of blood group A.
229. decreased in non-smokers compared with smokers.

Features of polycystic ovarian syndrome include

230. failure of follicular maturation.
231. elevated serum oestradiol concentrations.
232. elevated serum androstenedione concentrations.
233. endometrial hyperplasia.
234. breast atrophy.

An 18-year-old presents with secondary amenorrhoea following chemotherapy. The following diagnosis is likely:

235. polycystic ovarian syndrome.
236. weight-related amenorrhoea.
237. premature ovarian failure.
238. hyperprolactinaemia.

Concerning women taking hormone replacement therapy (HRT),

239. derivatives of 19-nortestosterone and medroxyprogesterone acetate produce similar changes in lipoprotein concentrations.
240. its use reduces the sensitivity of mammography for the detection of early malignant disease of the breast.
241. for diabetics it is not cardioprotective.
242. current use reduces mortality from cardiovascular disease by about 40%.
243. the increase in risk of breast cancer declines when treatment ceases.

Treatment with diethylstilboestrol in pregnancy has been shown to be associated with

244. an increased incidence of hypertensive disease of pregnancy.
245. oligozoospermia in the male offspring.
246. transverse bands in the vagina in the female offspring.

The serum luteinising hormone concentration is raised in

247. anorexia nervosa.
248. acromegaly.
249. polycystic ovarian syndrome.
250. cystadenocarcinoma of the ovary.

Concerning intrauterine insemination,

251. in unexplained infertility, live birth rates of greater than 20% per treatment can be obtained.
252. improved results are obtained when used in association with superovulation.
253. it should only be performed with washed and prepared sperm.
254. it is an effective treatment for oligozoospermic infertility.

In the male partner of an infertile couple,

255. azoospermia with a normal plasma follicle-stimulating hormone concentration indicates failure of the germinal epithelium.
256. oligozoospermia usually responds to treatment with androgens.

Recognised causes of erectile impotence in the male include

257. chronic renal failure.
258. sulfasalazine therapy.

Oocyte retrieval

259. is usually performed under general anaesthetic.
260. with aspiration of functional ovarian cysts prior to the treatment cycle results in increased oocyte yields.

Concerning the investigation of postmenopausal bleeding:

261. hysteroscopy is the most accurate means of assessment.
262. an endometrial thickness of less than 3 mm on transvaginal ultrasound makes endometrial sampling unnecessary.
263. on transvaginal ultrasound, colour Doppler imaging reliably differentiates benign from malignant lesions of the endometrium.
264. outpatient endometrial sampling is contraindicated.
265. a cervical smear should always be performed.

Premature ovarian failure in a woman aged 35 years can be diagnosed

266. after 12 months of amenorrhoea.
267. on the basis of sustained serum follicle-stimulating hormone concentrations of more than 50 iu/l.
268. by finding a monophasic basal body temperature.
269. on the basis of sustained high serum concentrations of androstenedione.

A 46-year-old woman has had an intrauterine contraceptive device (IUCD) in situ for a number of years. The following statements concerning her management are correct:

270. Changing the device increases the chance of her becoming pregnant.
271. If a copper bearing IUCD has been used for five years, it must be replaced.
272. If an inert IUCD has been used for ten years, it must be replaced.

Concerning the progestogen-only contraceptive pill,

273. extra contraceptive precautions should be used for at least 14 days if the pill is started on the first day of menstruation.
274. the development of amenorrhoea, in the absence of pregnancy, indicates anovulation.
275. its use confers some protection from sexually transmitted diseases.

The following statements concerning the fallopian tube are correct:

276. Pyosalpinx is a common sequel to post-abortion infection.
277. It is the commonest site for genital tuberculosis.

Recognised causes of postcoital bleeding include

278. cervical intraepithelial neoplasia stage 3 (CIN3).
279. an intrauterine contraceptive device.

Ovarian dermoid cysts (cystic teratomata) characteristically

280. arise principally from endodermal embryonal elements.
281. are bilateral in approximately 50% of cases.

Pseudomyxoma peritonei

282. requires leakage from a parent cyst for the development of the condition.
283. is characteristically associated with intestinal obstruction.
284. responds to treatment with alkylating agents.
285. is associated with pleural effusion.
286. is a complication of a ruptured mucocele of the appendix.

Recognised causes of cystic swellings within the female breast include

287. degeneration within a colloid carcinoma.
288. dysgerminoma of the ovary.
289. long-term use of the combined oral contraceptive.

Adrenal tumours causing female hirsutism are characteristically associated with

290. the absence of diurnal cortisol variation.
291. raised serum concentrations of adrenocorticotrophic hormone (ACTH).
292. raised serum 17-alpha-hydroxyprogesterone concentrations.

The following stages of malignant disease are correctly paired with the extent of the clinical spread described:

293. sage II carcinoma of the cervix : involvement of the lower third of the vagina.
294. stage III carcinoma of the ovary : widespread intraperitoneal metastases.
295. stage III carcinoma of the cervix : involvement of the rectal mucosa.
296. stage III carcinoma of the endometrium : involvement of the bladder mucosa.
297. stage III carcinoma of the endometrium : involvement of the rectal mucosa.

The following chemotherapeutic agents are characteristically associated with the stated side effects:

298. methotrexate: oral ulceration.
299. cisplatin: cardiotoxicity.
300. cyclophosphamide: ototoxicity.

March 1998

A recognised association exists between polyhydramnios and

1. anencephaly.
2. an imperforate anus in the fetus.
3. fetal polycystic kidneys.

The following have a recognised association with transverse lie of the fetus in late pregnancy or labour:

4. microcephaly.
5. high parity.
6. a bicornuate uterus.

Factors characteristically associated with the spontaneous onset of premature labour include

7. oligohydramnios.
8. urinary tract infection.
9. presence of vaginal group B haemolytic streptococcus.

The following statements concerning the bony pelvis are correct:

10. The angle of inclination of the pelvic brim is greater in Negroid than in Caucasian women.
11. In the anthropoid type of female pelvis, the anteroposterior diameter of the inlet is significantly greater than the transverse.
12. A straight sacrum is associated with a narrow subpubic angle.
13. The sacrosciatic notch is significantly wider in an android pelvis.
14. The female pelvis is characteristically shallower than the male pelvis.

The following are recognised to cross the placenta in clinically significant quantities:

15. indomethacin.
16. lithium.
17. cholestyramine.

18.   podophyllotoxin.
19.   propylthiouracil.

Amniocentesis

20.   carries an increased risk of orthopaedic deformity as a sequel.
21.   has a risk of chorioamnionitis in 3–5% of cases.

The following are recognised complications of the use of an intravenous oxytocin infusion:

22.   neonatal jaundice.
23.   maternal hyperglycaemia.

Compared with vacuum extraction, a Kielland forceps delivery is associated with an increased incidence of

24.   neonatal jaundice.
25.   subgaleal haematoma.
26.   facial palsy.

Congenital infection with cytomegalovirus

27.   is associated with intracerebral calcification.
28.   is associated with retarded fetal growth.
29.   is a recognised cause of microcephaly.
30.   can be detected by culture of the infant's urine.
31.   is associated with polyhydramnios.

Phaeochromocytoma complicating pregnancy is characteristically associated with

32.   secretion of dopamine.
33.   a high output of 5-hydroxyindole-acetic acid in the urine.
34.   impaired carbohydrate tolerance.
35.   precordial pain.

Disseminated intravascular coagulation has a recognised association with

36.   placenta praevia.
37.   multiple pregnancy.
38.   iron deficiency anaemia.
39.   prolonged bed rest.

Acute pulmonary thromboembolism occurring during pregnancy

40. has a recognised association with advancing maternal age.
41. is a recognised complication of severe iron deficiency anaemia.

Excess urobilinogen in the urine is a recognised feature of

42. cholestatic jaundice of pregnancy.
43. congenital spherocytosis.
44. sickle cell disease.
45. acute fatty liver.

Women with proteinuric pregnancy induced hypertension (pre-eclampsia) will characteristically show raised

46. creatinine clearance.
47. platelet concentration.

Asymptomatic bacteriuria in pregnancy

48. if untreated, is followed later in pregnancy by acute pyelonephritis in 60–70% of women.
49. is associated with raised levels of maternal serum alpha-fetoprotein at 16 weeks of gestation.

Patients with acute pyelonephritis in pregnancy

50. are at risk of developing endotoxic shock.

Regarding systemic lupus erythematosus in pregnancy:

51. In severe exacerbations of the disease, termination of pregnancy will usually lead to remission.
52. High levels of maternal antiphospholipid antibodies are associated with increased risk of pregnancy failure.
53. Fetal heart block occurs in at least 40% of babies.

The following statements regarding inflammatory bowel disease during pregnancy are correct:

54. In the acute phase of Crohn's disease in the first trimester of pregnancy, metronidazole is the treatment of choice.
55. Ulcerative colitis developing for the first time in pregnancy is likely to be severe.
56. Active Crohn's disease is commonly associated with megaloblastic anaemia.

57. Treatment with sulfasalazine is contraindicated.
58. Ulcerative colitis has a more than 50% chance of remaining quiescent.

The congenital rubella syndrome

59. can be prevented by the administration of immunoglobulin to an infected mother during pregnancy.
60. is associated with neonatal persistent ductus arteriosus.
61. includes neonatal purpura.
62. includes neonatal microcephaly.

The following are recognised effects of the administration of beta-agonists to the mother:

63. increased maternal pulse pressure.
64. decreased maternal blood insulin levels.

When pregnancy occurs in a woman over the age of 35 years, there is a recognised increase in

65. the incidence of pregnancy prolonged beyond 40 weeks.
66. the frequency of multiple pregnancy.
67. the frequency of fetal neural tube defects.
68. the incidence of placental abruption.
69. the incidence of fetal growth retardation.

In a child with Down syndrome there is a recognised association with

70. an atrial septal defect.
71. congenital duodenal atresia.
72. hypotonia.

The following diseases are inherited by autosomal recessive transmission:

73. Huntington's chorea.
74. myotonic dystrophy.
75. infantile polycystic kidneys.
76. galactosaemia.
77. achondroplasia.

The incidence of the following is increased in the preterm neonate:

78.   a patent ductus arteriosus.
79.   anaemia.
80.   meconium ileus.

Haemolytic disease of the newborn is

81.   characterised by erythroblasts in the cord blood.
82.   associated with a positive direct Coombs test in the cord blood.
83.   characterised by jaundice present at birth.
84.   associated with a prolonged prothrombin time.
85.   associated with persistence of the placental cytotrophoblast.

The following conditions would be expected to conform to the pattern of inheritance shown in Figure 2:

86.   polyposis coli.
87.   adrenal hyperplasia.
88.   haemophilia A (classical).
89.   congenital dislocation of the hip.

Congenital abnormalities in the fetus are more common after the following maternal infections during pregnancy:

90.   mumps.
91.   genital herpes simplex virus type II.
92.   malaria.
93.   toxoplasmosis.

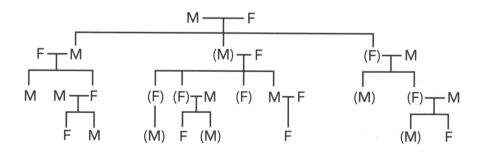

[M = normal male, (M) = affected male, F = normal female, (F) = carrier female]

Figure 2

The following disorders are correctly associated with the mode of inheritance:

94. von Recklinghausen's disease (neurofibromatosis) : autosomal dominant.
95. Tay-Sach's disease : autosomal recessive.

Sacral agenesis

96. is a recognised complication of propylthiouracil treatment in the first trimester.
97. is a recognised complication of fetal toxoplasmosis.
98. has an association with an elevated maternal serum alpha-fetoprotein level.
99. is related to poor glucose homeostasis in the first trimester.

The following statements concerning fetal hydrocephalus are correct:

100. chromosomal abnormalities are found in less than 15% of cases.
101. it has a causal association with fetal viral infections.
102. it may be a result of Arnold–Chiari malformation.

With regard to anencephaly,

103. small adrenal glands are characteristic.
104. the midbrain is absent.
105. renal agenesis is commonly associated.

Maternal administration of glucocorticoids used to prevent respiratory distress syndrome in the newborn

106. is contraindicated between 26 and 32 weeks of gestation in the presence of ruptured membranes.
107. is most effective if given within 48 hours before delivery.
108. suppresses neonatal adrenal function.
109. has not been shown to reduce the incidence of the condition.

Regarding the fetal heart,

110. More than 10% of fetuses with persistent antepartum bradycardia have a structural cardiac abnormality.
111. 80% of late decelerations in labour are associated with a pH of less than 7.20.
112. Fetal heart pulsation can be seen at five weeks (after the last menstrual period) on vaginal scan.

Duchenne muscular dystrophy

113. may be identified by measuring the maternal creatine kinase activity at 18 weeks of gestation.
114. is the most common X-linked cause of reduced life expectancy in males.
115. only occurs when the mother carries the defective gene.
116. may now be effectively treated with the protein 'dystrophin'.

For a pregnant woman, the risk of having a fetus affected by Down syndrome

117. that is born at term is, at a maternal age of thirty-five years, approximately 1/360 births.
118. increases if serum beta-human chorionic gonadotrophin concentration is elevated at 16 weeks of pregnancy.
119. increases if the woman has had a previous child with Down syndrome.
120. is increased if a single stomach bubble is identified on ultrasound examination.
121. at ten weeks is approximately double that of having an affected live baby.

With regard to non-immune hydrops fetalis,

122. if the condition is detected antenatally, delivery should be by caesarean section.
123. it may be caused by intrauterine acquired infection.
124. there is a 20% risk of chromosomal abnormality.

Drugs considered suitable to be prescribed to the breastfeeding mother include

125. phenytoin.
126. mefenamic acid.
127. propylthiouracil.

Breastfeeding is compromised by

128. dopamine agonists.
129. metronidazole.
130. metoclopramide.
131. depo-medroxyprogesterone acetate.

The following conditions and features occurring in pregnancy are appropriately paired:

132. mitral stenosis : orthopnoea.
133. hyperthyroidism : acne.
134. Hodgkin's disease : fever.

In a prospective blind study of a possible new method of antenatal screening for a particular fetal disorder, 60 000 consecutive pregnant women were recruited and tested. One hundred of the fetuses were found to be affected. The test had a sensitivity of 90% and a specificity of 95%. Based on this study the following statements are correct:

135. A woman with a positive test has a 10% chance of having an affected child.
136. The results demonstrate that the test fulfils the criteria set by the World Health Organization for screening.
137. 95% of affected cases had a positive screening test.
138. The false positive rate can be calculated using Fisher's exact test.

With regard to premature ovarian failure,

139. it should be differentiated from resistant ovarian syndrome by ovarian biopsy.
140. serum concentrations of follicle-stimulating hormone greater than 40 iu/l indicate permanent ovarian failure.
141. it is associated with an increased risk of ovarian malignancy.
142. it is usually associated with an identifiable autoimmune factor.
143. it increases the risk of myocardial infarction.

Changes in the serum compatible with a premature menopause include

144. an increase in prolactin concentration.
145. an increase in calcium levels.
146. an increase in cholesterol levels.
147. an increase in free testosterone levels.

Characteristic features of the androgen insensitivity (testicular feminisation) syndrome in an adult include

148. a family history of the condition.
149. absence of axillary hair.
150. the 47XXY karyotype.
151. breast hypoplasia.

152. hypospadias.

Secondary amenorrhoea is a recognised feature of

153. Addison's disease.
154. chronic renal failure.
155. beta-thalassaemia major.
156. Down syndrome.
157. bulimia.

Precocious puberty

158. of the constitutional type has a familial incidence in approximately 45% of cases.
159. of the constitutional type is more common in boys than in girls.
160. is a recognised feature of polyostotic fibrous dysplasia (Albright's syndrome).
161. has a recognised association with benign teratoma of the ovary.
162. has a recognised association with juvenile hypothyroidism.

In patients with Turner syndrome,

163. pregnancy may be achieved by assisted conception using donated ova.
164. uterine bleeding can be induced with cyclical oestrogen/progesterone therapy.
165. oestrogen therapy to induce puberty should be delayed if treatment with growth hormone is to be offered.
166. breast development will be poor.

A thirty-year-old woman 1.6 m in height complains of secondary amenorrhoea and 'hot flushes'. Her periods began at the age of 12 years and were regular until eight months ago, when they stopped suddenly. After the birth of her second child (six years ago) she had a postpartum haemorrhage, necessitating a three-unit blood transfusion. Four years ago, she was diagnosed as having insulin-dependent diabetes, which has been difficult to control. As a result of this and her husband's unemployment she has lost 7 kg to her present weight of 45 kg (body mass index 17.59). Her blood chemistry results include: 17-beta oestradiol 80 pmol/l; follicle-stimulating hormone 44 iu/l; cortisol 130 nmol/l. On the information given above, the following statements are correct:

167. Weight gain of about 5 kg will almost certainly lead to a return of menstruation.

168. Successful stabilisation of her diabetes is likely to result in a return of menstruation.
169. The clinical picture is consistent with autoimmune ovarian failure.
170. Without treatment she is at risk of developing premature osteoporosis.
171. A diagnosis of panhypopituitarism has not been excluded.

Recognised causes of galactorrhoea include

172. primary hypothyroidism.
173. pituitary stalk section.
174. chronic renal failure.
175. administration of spironolactone.
176. herpes zoster of the intercostal nerves.

In a patient with inappropriate lactation associated with secondary amenorrhoea,

177. bi-temporal hemianopia on perimetry would be expected in about 25% of patients.
178. an increased plasma progesterone concentration would be expected.
179. the administration of methyldopa is a recognised cause.
180. anorexia nervosa is a recognised association.

With regard to the finding of a pelvic mass in an adolescent girl,

181. there is a recognised association between gonadal dysgenesis and a dysgerminoma.
182. subsequent ultrasound assessment showing a solid ovarian tumour is suggestive of a dysgerminoma.
183. the diagnosis of haematocolpos may be made clinically.
184. the most common type of ovarian cyst is an epithelial cystadenoma.

Azoospermia associated with high levels of follicle-stimulating hormone is characteristically found in the presence of

185. Klinefelter syndrome.
186. testicular atrophy.
187. congenital absence of the vas deferens.
188. bilateral varicocele.
189. a previous vasectomy.

Oligozoospermia has a recognised association with

190. bronchiectasis.
191. sulfasalazine therapy.

Sperm transport through the cervical canal may be impaired by

192. the presence of Escherichia coli in the cervical mucus.
193. the preovulatory surge of luteinising hormone.
194. clomifene citrate.

Recognised effects of progestogen-only oral contraceptive therapy include

195. inhibition of ovulation in over 90% of subjects.
196. poor cycle control.
197. fibroadenosis of the breast.
198. intrahepatic cholestasis.

The following statements relating to sexual dysfunction are correct:

199. A complaint of recurrent vaginal discharge, with no detectable pathology, is a recognised presentation of psychosexual difficulties.
200. Patients with psychosexual problems commonly have a psychiatric illness.
201. A past history of sexual abuse is commonly found.
202. Frequently, both partners will have a sexual problem.

Procedures of value in the diagnosis of acute gonorrhoea in the female include

203. culture of a high vaginal swab.
204. a complement fixation test.
205. the naked-eye examination of the vaginal discharge.
206. culture of a swab from the anal canal.

The toxic shock syndrome has a recognised association with

207. a fever of 39°C or more.
208. diarrhoea.
209. a generalised macular erythema.
210. isolation of the group B streptococcus.

Enterocele

211. is characteristically associated with difficulty in emptying the rectum.
212. can be congenital.
213. is a recognised complication of vaginal hysterectomy.
214. is characteristically associated with painful defaecation.

Genuine stress incontinence of urine is characteristically

215. associated with laxity of the pubourethral ligaments.
216. improves during pregnancy.
217. caused by an overactive detrusor muscle.
218. can only be diagnosed by urodynamic investigation.
219. improved by elevation of the urethrovesical angle.

Features characteristically associated with an imperforate vagina in a girl aged 16 years include

220. absence of secondary sexual characteristics.
221. an XX karyotype.
222. a pelvic kidney.
223. short stature.
224. closed spina bifida.

Pyometra is a recognised complication of

225. acute endometritis.
226. cone biopsy of the cervix.
227. intrauterine contraceptive devices.

The following statements concerning trophoblastic disease are correct:

228. Choriocarcinoma may be accompanied by clinical evidence of thyrotoxicosis.
229. There is a significant increase in incidence beyond the age of 40 years.
230. The prognosis is influenced by the patient's ABO blood group.
231. The tissue karyotype is characteristically 46XX.

Characteristic features of primary spasmodic dysmenorrhoea include

232. relief of pain by mefenamic acid.
233. a delayed menarche.

234. raised concentrations of serum prolactin.
235. an association with uterine hypoplasia.

Noninvasive (complete) hydatidiform mole

236. has a ten times increased risk of occurring in a subsequent pregnancy compared with women who have no history of molar pregnancy.
237. occurs most frequently in a first pregnancy.
238. occurs in less than 1.5/1000 pregnancies in Western Europe.

The following predispose to the development of endometrial carcinoma:

239. adrenal hyperplasia.
240. tamoxifen therapy.
241. polycystic ovary syndrome.

Endometrial hyperplasia is characteristically associated with

242. anovulatory cycles.
243. hyperthyroidism.
244. vaginal adenosis.
245. hyperprolactinaemia.
246. the use of intrauterine contraceptive devices.

Uterine curettage

247. is essential in the investigation of secondary amenorrhoea.
248. is curative in about 50% of cases of menorrhagia of unknown aetiology.

In women with objectively measured idiopathic heavy menstrual bleeding

249. there is abnormal platelet function in the uterine blood vessels.
250. treatment with a levonorgestrel-releasing intrauterine system leads to a greater than 70% reduction in blood loss within six months.

In the international classification (FIGO) of ovarian carcinoma

251. stage II carcinoma is limited to the ovaries.
252. secondary deposits in the omentum indicate stage III.
253. ascites can be present in stage I.
254. a pleural effusion with negative cytology indicates stage III.

Ovarian tumours which secrete oestrogens include

255. thecoma.
256. serous cystadenoma.
257. dysgerminoma.
258. granulosa cell tumour.

Bilateral oophorectomy in premenopausal women

259. is indicated at the time of radical hysterectomy for cervical cancer in young women.
260. should be performed at the time of hysterectomy for fibroids in women aged 40 years.
261. is associated with an increased incidence of coronary heart disease.
262. is required in women under the age of 30 years who have stage Ia ovarian cancer.
263. is indicated in patients with XO gonadal dysgenesis.

Krukenberg tumours

264. contain Kupffer cells.
265. are characteristically bilateral.
266. characteristically occur after the menopause.

Ovarian neoplasms occurring under the age of 20 years

267. require the removal of the contralateral ovary if a malignant germ-cell tumour is diagnosed.
268. are most commonly epithelial in type.

Ovarian thecomas

269. are typically benign.
270. are characteristically bilateral.
271. characteristically occur before puberty.
272. are a recognised cause of pseudo-Meig syndrome.
273. may present with virilising symptoms.

Cisplatin

274. usually causes alopecia.
275. is ototoxic.
276. seldom produces severe myelosuppression.

Noncystic lesions of the vulva include

277. hidradenoma.
278. accessory breast tissue.
279. Nabothian follicles.

Recognised causes of vulval ulceration include

280. lymphogranuloma venereum (*Chlamydia trachomatis*).
281. lichen sclerosus.
282. Behçet's syndrome.
283. tuberculosis.
284. actinomycosis.

Routine examination of a cervical smear can identify the presence of

285. *Trichomonas vaginalis.*
286. *Chlamydia trachomatis.*
287. *Neisseria gonorrhoea.*
288. *Candida albicans.*

The following are correctly paired with a recognised clinical association:

289. carcinoma of ovary : hypocalcaemia
290. inappropriate secretion of antidiuretic hormone : hypernatraemia
291. retroperitoneal sarcoma : diabetes mellitus
292. uterine fibroids : polycythaemia
293. adrenal carcinoma : hirsutism

The following disorders are correctly linked with a recognised association:

294. polycystic ovary disease : raised serum sex hormone-binding globulin.
295. isolated gonadotrophin deficiency : anosmia.
296. pure gonadal dysgenesis : 46XY karyotype.
297. androgen insensitivity syndrome : hirsutism.
298. Klinefelter syndrome : impotence.

The following conditions are correctly paired with a characteristic laboratory finding:

299. constitutional (idiopathic) hirsutism : elevated serum sex hormone-binding globulin.
300. anorexia nervosa : elevated serum follicle-stimulating hormone.

September 1998

The following statements relating to pregnancy in a 38-year-old woman are correct:

F 1. Her risk of a child with neural-tube defect is ten times greater than at the age of eighteen years.

F 2. Chorionic villus biopsy will allow diagnosis of neural-tube defect.

T 3. Her risk of a child with Down syndrome is less than 1%.

Down syndrome

T 4. has an incidence in the United Kingdom of approximately one in 700 live births.

F 5. is more commonly due to translocation than to nondisjunction.

The following disorders are correctly associated with their mode of inheritance:

T 6. glucose-6-phosphate dehydrogenase deficiency : X-linked recessive.

F 7. polycystic disease of kidneys (adult form) : multifactorial.

T 8. von Willebrand's disease : autosomal dominant.

Methods of value to distinguish the fetus with intrauterine growth restriction from that of uncertain gestational age include

T 9. increasing ratio of head to abdominal circumference measured by ultrasound.

F 10. measurement of fetal breathing activity.

F 11. cardiac volume.

Recognised causes of nonimmunological hydrops fetalis include

T 12. cytomegalovirus infection.

T 13. alpha-thalassaemia.

F 14. renal agenesis.

An increased risk of fetal malformation is associated with

F 15. the presence of a single umbilical vein.
F 16. smoking 20 cigarettes or more a day.
? T 17. rubella vaccination in the first trimester of pregnancy.

The fetal alcohol syndrome

F 18. is associated with an increased incidence of postmaturity.
T 19. seldom occurs with alcohol ingestion by the mother of under eight units per week (one unit = one glass of wine).
F 20. is reversed by a high intake of vitamins.

A geneticist notices with concern that a striking similarity in appearance exists between his son and a male neighbour. The geneticist would be reassured that he, and not the neighbour, is the true father of the child if

F 21. the neighbour and the son have a normal but unusual polymorphic variant of chromosome 9.
? F 22. the neighbour's blood group is A rhesus positive and the son's is B rhesus negative.
? T 23. the neighbour has cystic fibrosis.

The administration of corticosteroids is appropriate management in those pregnancies that are affected by:

T 24. hyperemesis gravidarum.
T 25. triplets.
T 26. systemic lupus erythematosus.

A woman presents at 38 weeks of gestation with right iliac fossa pain. Likely causes include

F 27. acute salpingitis.
T 28. a strangulated inguinal hernia.
T 29. constipation.

Recognised complications of fibroids during pregnancy include

F 30. placenta accreta.
F 31. precipitate labour.
? F 32. fetal growth restriction.

Factors favouring placental abruption include

F 33. von Willebrand's disease.
F 34. pregnancy associated with an intrauterine contraceptive device.

Complications of placental abruption include

T 35. postpartum haemorrhage.
F 36. folic acid deficiency.

The following statements regarding a parous, rhesus negative, unsensitised woman who is pregnant by a new partner who is rhesus positive (D-heterozygous) are correct:

T 37. Group O Rhesus negative blood crossmatched against the mother's serum should be used if intrafetal transfusion is indicated.
T 38. There is a 50% chance that her baby will be rhesus negative.

In a woman with a primary cytomegalovirus (CMV) infection in pregnancy,

T 39. there is a less than 5% chance of her delivering a baby with CMV-related damage.
T 40. there is a 1% chance of the baby having serious long-term sequelae.
F 41. antenatal treatment reduces the risk of neonatal complications.

The following statements regarding toxoplasmosis are correct:

T 42. The incidence of toxoplasma infections in pregnant women in the UK is about 2/1000 pregnancies.
T 43. Spiramycin is used in the treatment of *in utero* toxoplasma infections.
F 44. *Toxoplasma gondii* is a cause of repeated miscarriage.

The following maternal infections may be transmitted to the newborn as a result of vaginal delivery:

T 45. herpes simplex virus.
T 46. human papillomavirus.
T 47. *Trichomonas vaginalis*.

In patients with HIV infection

F 48. the rate of transmission to the fetus in a seropositive mother is over 50%.

T 49. a recognised presentation is *Pneumocystis carinii* pneumonia.
F 50. pregnancy may accelerate the development of AIDS in seropositive women.

A 24-year-old woman is seen at the antenatal clinic in the tenth week of her second pregnancy. She reports that, one week previously, her two-year-old daughter had a generalised skin rash which had been diagnosed as rubella. The patient has no memory of herself having had German measles. Serological testing confirms the presence of rubella antibodies at a low titre of 1:8. From this information, the following statements are true:

F 51. Pooled immunoglobulin should be given if maternal infection is suspected.
T 52. Congenital anomalies in an affected fetus include cataract.
F 53. The serological test result confirms recent maternal infection.
T 54. The test should be repeated in the following week.

Pregnancy exacerbates the clinical features associated with

F 55. sarcoidosis.
T 56. sickle cell haemoglobinopathy.
T 57. cutaneous neurofibromatosis.
F 58. von Willebrand's disease.
F 59. coeliac disease.

The following statements concerning drug therapy in severe pregnancy-induced hypertension are correct:

F 60. Treatment with methyldopa should be limited to dosages of less than 2 g per day.
T 61. Headache is a recognised side effect of hydralazine.
T 62. Labetalol is a combined alpha- and beta-adrenergic blocking agent.
T 63. Nifedipine has a rapid onset of action.

The following statements about drug treatment in eclampsia are correct:

T 64. Maternal administration of intravenous diazepam characteristically causes diminution of fetal heart rate variation.
T 65. Neonatal respiratory depression is a recognised complication of magnesium sulphate overdosage.
T 66. Magnesium sulphate may be administered by the intramuscular route.

Regarding peripartum cardiomyopathy,

T 67. cerebral embolisation is a major cause of morbidity.
F 68. cardiac transplantation is inappropriate.
F 69. the mortality rate within the first year is greater than 80%.
T 70. anticoagulation is required.

The following statements regarding epilepsy complicating pregnancy are correct:

T 71. Pregnant women with a history of epilepsy who do not require anticonvulsant therapy have an increased risk of fetal malformation.
F 72. Breastfeeding is contraindicated in women taking anticonvulsants.

The following complications of pregnancy or the puerperium are correctly paired:

T 73. sickle cell disease : pregnancy-induced hypertension.
T 74. chorioangioma of the placenta : polyhydramnios.
T 75. eclampsia : thrombocytopenia.

In pregnancy complicated by insulin-dependent maternal diabetes mellitus

T 76. the risk of intrauterine death of the fetus is greatest during the last four weeks of pregnancy.
T 77. the insulin requirement may decrease during the first trimester.
T 78. a normal HbAl level is associated with a low risk of fetal abnormality.

In sickle cell disease associated with pregnancy

T 79. maternal mortality (in the UK) is of the order of 1% of affected mothers.
F 80. vitamin C supplements should be given.
T 81. iron deficiency is rare.

In relation to monozygotic (uniovular) twin pregnancy

T 82. 'situs inversus' occurs more commonly in a monozygotic twin than in the general population.
T 83. the incidence is approximately 25% of all twin pregnancies.
T 84. acute polyhydramnios is more common than in dizygotic twin pregnancy.

External cephalic version after 37 completed weeks of gestation

T 85. is a recognised cause of fetal bradycardia.
F 86. is likely to lead to transient maternal hypertension.
F 87. should only be performed using tocolytic agents.
T 88. is successful in over 25% of cases.

The following drugs, administered in therapeutic dosage during the third trimester of pregnancy, are correctly paired with a recognised adverse effect in the fetus or neonate:

T 89. labetalol : neonatal hypoglycaemia.
? T 90. lithium carbonate : respiratory distress syndrome.
? T 91. phenytoin : coagulation defects.

The following are characteristically associated with spontaneous preterm delivery:

T 92. cocaine abuse throughout pregnancy.
T 93. placental chorioangioma.
F 94. placental sulphatase deficiency.

The following statements relating to premature labour are correct:

T 95. Beta-sympathomimetic agents used in conjunction with corticosteroids in premature labour are a recognised cause of maternal pulmonary oedema.
F 96. Premature rupture of the membranes is frequently consequent upon orgasm.

The following statements relating to the use of prostaglandins (PG) are correct:

F 97. PGE_2 0.5 mg vaginally will induce labour in 80% of women with an unripe cervix.
F 98. $PGF2\alpha$ is ten times more potent than PGE_2 in inducing contractions.
T 99. Beta-agonists will suppress the contractions induced by prostaglandins.

The umbilical cord

F 100. is more likely to prolapse if greater than 35 cm in length.
F 101. vessels require fetoscopic visualisation prior to cordocentesis.
T 102. absorbs water from the umbilical fluid.

Early decelerations in the fetal heart rate in labour

F 103. are a sign of fetal hypoxia.
F 104. indicate fetal distress if they occur repeatedly.

Spinal analgesia (subarachnoid block) in obstetric practice

F 105. is not suitable as an anaesthetic in the manual removal of a retained placenta.
T 106. reduces the incidence of perioperative shivering compared with epidural analgesia.
F 107. is associated with less hypotension than with epidural analgesia.

Following vaginal delivery of the first twin,

F 108. the fetal heart rate should be noted after each contraction.
F 109. internal podalic version is no longer an acceptable procedure.

Predisposing factors to face presentation include

T 110. sternomastoid tumour.
T 111. contracted pelvis.
T 112. preterm labour.

The following statements regarding occipitoposterior (OP) positions are correct:

T 113. Between 10% and 20% of all cephalic presentations are occipitoposterior in early labour.
T 114. Less than 10% will deliver spontaneously face-to-pubis.
T 115. Labour is associated with early spontaneous rupture of the membranes.
F 116. In multiparous women, it is the commonest cause of a high head at term.

A randomised double-blinded trial was conducted on the use of suture materials X and Y for repairing episiotomies, with the addition of an oral anti-inflammatory compound or a placebo. The outcome of the trial was measured by the need for analgesic drugs and the table shows the proportion of women in the four treatment groups who required an analgesic on the second postpartum day.

Treatment group	Proportion needing analgesia
1. Suture X + anti-inflammatory drug	27/42 (64.3%) = 51/84 (60.7%)
2. Suture X + placebo	24/42 (57.1%)
3. Suture Y + anti-inflammatory drug	22/42 (52.4%) = 48/88 (54.5%)
4. Suture Y + placebo	26/46 (56.5%)

The following statements are correct:

F   117. In the comparison of suture X with suture Y, if $P = 0.4$ then the result observed would have occurred by chance on four occasions out of 1000.

F   118. The superiority of suture Y over suture X has been statistically proven.

T   119. Chi-squared is an appropriate statistical test to analyse these data.

In amniotic fluid embolism,

F   120. detection of trophoblastic cells in the peripheral circulation is pathognomonic.

F   121. the patient is likely to be a primigravida.

F   122. 25% of fatalities occur within one hour of the onset of symptoms.

In the management of massive haemorrhage in the labour ward,

T   123. if additional calcium is needed, then 10% calcium gluconate should be given.

T   124. blood should be administered through blood-warming equipment.

F   125. platelet concentrates should be transfused at an early stage.

Recognised features of massive central pulmonary embolism include

F   126. clinical evidence of deep venous thrombosis in the lower limb in more than 60% of patients.

F   127. pulmonary vascular congestion on the chest X-ray.

T   128. sinus tachycardia.

Acute inversion of the uterus

T 129. occurs most commonly when the placenta is sited in the fundus of the uterus.

F 130. is more common in twin than single pregnancy.

Blood loss of more than 500 ml within 12 hours of the delivery of the placenta has a recognised association with

T 131. a low implantation site of the placenta.

T 132. Couvelaire uterus.

T 133. halothane anaesthesia.

F 134. beta-thalassaemia.

The following statements referring to mortality statistics within the UK are correct:

F 135. Perinatal mortality is defined as the sum of stillbirths and neonatal deaths occurring in the first 28 days of life for each 1000 live births.

T 136. A neonatal death is defined as the death of an infant born alive and who dies within 28 days, irrespective of the stage of gestation.

F 137. A late neonatal death is defined as a death between 14 and 28 days.

F 138. Infant mortality excludes deaths in the first month of life.

F 139. A stillbirth is defined as an infant born dead and weighing over 1000 g.

In relation to lactation, the following statements are correct:

T 140. Only colostrum is produced at the time of delivery.

F 141. Breast engorgement occurs during the first 24 hours following delivery.

When compared with bottle feeding, breast feeding is associated with a decreased risk of

T 142. sudden infant death syndrome.

T 143. atopic eczema.

T 144. necrotising enterocolitis.

The perinatal mortality rate is significantly increased by the following maternal factors:

F 145. chickenpox (varicella) in early pregnancy.

T 146. systemic lupus erythematosus in pregnancy.

The incidence of neonatal respiratory distress syndrome is characteristically increased

F 147. in full term infants born below the tenth centile for birth weight.
T 148. following prolonged intrauterine hypoxia.

Necrotising enterocolitis is characterised by

T 149. blood in the stool.
T 150. bile-stained vomit.

The following pairs of items are causally linked:

T 151. tracheo-oesophageal fistula : polyhydramnios.
F 152. hypercalcaemia : neonatal convulsions.
T 153. imperforate anus : polyhydramnios.

Recognised associations exist between mid-trimester miscarriage and

F 154. beta-thalassaemia.
T 155. bleeding in the first trimester.
T 156. death of one fetus in a twin pregnancy.

Characteristic features of hydatidiform mole include

F 157. bilateral follicular cysts.
F 158. an XY chromosomal karyotype.
T 159. an increased incidence in women over the age of 40 years.

When prostaglandins are used alone for the termination of pregnancy they are associated with

F 160. an induction–abortion interval in the second trimester of under 12 hours in more than 50% of cases.
T 161. hypertension.
F 162. an antidiuretic effect.

The following statements concerning legal termination of pregnancy in England and Wales are correct:

F 163. The signatures of two registered medical practitioners, one of whom must be a qualified gynaecologist, are required.
F 164. Rhesus prophylaxis is unnecessary when termination is before eight weeks.

A two-year-old girl has a persistent vaginal discharge that causes vulval irritation and staining of her underwear. The following statements are correct:

T 165. When the discharge is blood stained, an examination under anaesthesia is required.

F 166. Broad-spectrum antibiotics are the treatment of choice.

T 167. Sexual abuse should be considered as a cause.

F 168. Most cases are characterised by recurrence until puberty.

Recognised associations of abnormal uterine development include

T 169. acute retention of urine.

T 170. primary infertility.

T 171. the presence of a pelvic kidney.

Recognised associations of oligomenorrhoea include

T 172. chronic renal failure.

T 173. cystic glandular hyperplasia of the endometrium.

Concerning premature ovarian failure presenting as secondary amenorrhoea in a woman aged 30 years,

T 174. less than 10% have a chromosomal aetiology.

T 175. it is clinically indistinguishable from resistant ovarian syndrome.

F 176. over 30% have an autoimmune aetiology.

Uterine fibroids

F 177. are the most common site of leiomyosarcoma development.

F 178. if small and submucous are unlikely to be associated with menorrhagia.

F 179. can be accurately located by pelvic ultrasound.

F 180. if palpable abdominally should be removed.

Recognised causes of galactorrhoea include

T 181. acromegaly.

T 182. therapy with methyldopa.

T 183. hypothyroidism.

Women with polycystic ovary syndrome are more likely than women with normal ovaries

T 184. if oligomenorrhoeic to achieve a regular cycle by weight reduction alone.
T 185. to have an atherogenic lipid profile.
T 186. to have an elevated plasma testosterone concentration.
T 187. to be hyperinsulinaemic.

A twenty-four-year old woman complains of recent growth of excessive facial and limb hair. Menstruation is normal. Examination confirms the presence of normal breast development, external genitalia and pelvic organs. In relation to this patient, the following statements are correct:

? F 188. If all biochemical tests are normal, treatment with cyproterone acetate is indicated.
T 189. Investigation should include pelvic ultrasound.

Obesity is associated with an increased incidence of

T 190. thromboembolic disease.
T 191. endometrial carcinoma.
F 192. squamous carcinoma of the cervix.

Isolated gonadotrophin deficiency (Kallman syndrome)

F 193. is due to failure of development of the gonadotrophin producing cells of the pituitary.
F 194. is a recognised cause of secondary amenorrhoea.
T 195. has a recognised association with anosmia.

The following drugs are correctly paired with the side effects indicated:

T 196. mefenamic acid : diarrhoea.
? F 197. salazopyrine : impotence.
T 198. oxybutynin hydrochloride : dryness of the mouth.

Acute trichomoniasis in women of reproductive age is characterised by

F 199. a bloodstained vaginal discharge.
F 200. vulval oedema and fissure formation.
F 201. recent ingestion of a broad-spectrum antibiotic.

The following statements regarding genital herpes are correct:

202. The acquisition of herpes simplex virus (HSV) type 1 offers some protection against HSV type II infection.
203. acyclovir treatment significantly reduces the recrudescence rate.

A 20-year-old married woman presents with a history of offensive irritant vaginal discharge. She has taken a low-dose combined oral contraceptive pill for the last six months. Examination reveals an inflamed cervix and vagina with an offensive discharge. The uterus is anteverted and normal in size but there is general tenderness on pelvic examination. The following statements, relating to this history, are correct:

204. A negative high vaginal culture excludes gonococcal infection.
205. The signs and symptoms are highly suggestive of cervical ectopy.

The following statements relating to patients with psychosexual problems are correct:

206. Successful treatment of vaginismus includes Faradic stimulation of the pelvic floor.
207. There is an underlying psychiatric illness in the majority of patients.
208. A past history of sexual abuse is commonly found.

If a woman has an increased menstrual flow associated with an intrauterine device, the following statements are correct:

209. Her total blood loss can be reduced by over 50% by using mefenamic acid 500 mg three times a day.
210. The volume of bleeding is directly associated with the size of the device.
211. Antifibrinolytic agents are of therapeutic value.

The following statements relating to the progestogen-only oral contraceptive are correct:

212. Endometrial decidualisation occurs.
213. Lactation is inhibited.
214. There is an increase in the incidence of functional ovarian cysts.

In a woman taking a combined oral contraceptive preparation

215. the risk of impaired glucose tolerance rises with increasing age.
216. there is an increased risk of subarachnoid haemorrhage.

With regard to female sterilisation as practised in the UK,

T 217. there is an increased failure rate if performed at the same time as termination of pregnancy.
F 218. the consent of the partner is mandatory.
T 219. it is the commonest contraception used by those whose family is complete.

The following conditions are correctly paired with an appropriate treatment:

F 220. primary ovarian failure : clomifene citrate.
T 221. Central (true) precocious puberty : gonadotrophin-releasing hormone analogue.

Medroxyprogesterone acetate

T 222. is an effective contraceptive agent.
T 223. is associated with breakthrough bleeding.
F 224. suppresses lactation.

Gonadotrophin-releasing hormone agonists

F 225. when used in the treatment of endometriosis require pulsatile administration.
T 226. can be used simultaneously with hormone replacement therapy as appropriate therapy for endometriosis.

A 23-year-old woman married for three years complains of primary infertility and amenorrhoea since discontinuing oral contraceptive therapy one year ago. While taking oral contraception her weight increased from 60.8 kg (134 lbs) to 74.4 kg (164 lbs). Her height is 164 cm (5 feet 6 inches) and general systematic and pelvic examinations reveal no abnormality. A diagnostic test for pregnancy carried out on a specimen of urine one week previously was negative. Relevant further investigations include

T 227. serum prolactin estimation.
F 228. serial serum oestradiol estimations.

Concerning the use of clomifene citrate,

F 229. It will induce ovulation in women with weight-related amenorrhoea.
T 230. When used alone it is associated with the development of ovarian hyperstimulation syndrome.

An initial abnormal seminal analysis requires the following further measures:

F 231. referral for urological investigation.
F 232. the administration of testosterone proprionate.

Concerning *in vitro* fertilisation,

T 233. the age of the patient influences the pregnancy rate independent of the number of oocytes recovered.
F 234. in the UK the replacement of more than three embryos is permitted in exceptional circumstances.
F 235. oocyte recovery should be attempted within 24 hours of human chorionic gonadotrophin administration.

The following statements relating to the menopause are correct:

F 236. Frequency of micturition is a characteristic symptom.
F 237. Atrophic change in the vagina commonly presents with pruritus.
F 238. Obese women are more symptomatic than thin women.

Hormone replacement therapy for the postmenopausal woman is associated with

F 239. a decrease in the concentrations of factor VIII.
T 240. a decrease in the concentrations of serum follicle-stimulating hormone.
T 241. an increased incidence of coronary artery disease.

Recognised features of pelvic endometriosis include

T 242. an association with low fertility.
F 243. anovulatory cycles.
T 244. painful defaecation.

Conventional urodynamic studies (dual-channel subtracted cystometry with simultaneous pressure–flow measurements) are essential to distinguish between

F 245. patients with genuine stress incontinence who would best be treated by surgery and those where physiotherapy is indicated.
F 246. bacterial cystitis and interstitial cystitis.
T 247. detrusor instability and impaired compliance.

Factors which predispose to urinary tract infection include

T   248. postmenopausal vaginitis.

T   249. renal calculus.

Subsequent genital prolapse may be prevented by

F   250. elective induction of labour at term.

? T 251. continuing hormone replacement therapy.

The following statements concerning vulval disorders are correct:

T   252. Paget's disease is associated with apocrine carcinoma.

F   253. Lichen sclerosus should be treated by simple vulvectomy.

An acute tubo-ovarian abscess is associated with

T   254. diarrhoea.

T   255. bacteraemia.

T   256. a recognisable swelling on ultrasound examination.

Regarding the management of a patient after initial treatment for cervical intraepithelial neoplasia,

T   257. The incidence of dyskaryosis is greater if papillomavirus (HPV) infection had been present at the time of initial treatment.

T   258. The risk of invasive cervical cancer occurring is about five times that of the general population.

T   259. Women should have annual smears for ten years before returning to the general screening programme.

T   260. Vault smears should be taken for five years after hysterectomy.

F   261. Treatment reduces an individual's risk of invasive cancer by about 95%.

Loop diathermy for the management of cervical intraepithelial neoplasia

F   262. utilises a low current to enable an adequate histological interpretation of the excised tissue.

T   263. may be performed at any time during the menstrual cycle.

Carcinoma of the uterine cervix

T   264. characteristically originates from the transformation zone.

F   265. stage II is commonly associated with ureteric obstruction.

T   266. is an adenocarcinoma in between 10% and 20% of cases.

Recognised associations of endometrial hyperplasia include

T 267. essential hypertension.
F 268. prolonged postpartum anovulation.

Endometrial carcinoma

F 269. is histologically well differentiated in the majority of cases.
F 270. has metastasised to the ovaries in approximately 30% of cases at presentation.
F 271. characteristically causes intermenstrual bleeding.

With regard to leiomyosarcoma of the uterus,

T 272. recurrence of disease occurs in more than 50% of cases.
T 273. it carries a better prognosis in premenopausal than in postmenopausal women.
T 274. adjuvant pelvic irradiation does not improve survival.

Benign cystic teratomata (dermoid) of the ovary characteristically

F 275. are associated with menorrhagia.
T 276. have cells containing Barr bodies.
F 277. are multilocular.
T 278. are lined by squamous epithelium.

An ovarian tumour

F 279. when malignant has a significantly improved prognosis if a cytotoxic drug is instilled into the peritoneal cavity at the time of laparotomy.
T 280. undergoes torsion as a recognised complication.
F 281. if primary is characterised by the presence of signet-ring cells.

The following statements concerning epithelial ovarian cancer in the UK are correct:

T 282. Prophylactic bilateral oophorectomy at the time of hysterectomy would prevent about 10% of all cases.
F 283. Second-look laparotomy is justified by an improved five-year survival rate.
F 284. It is associated with prolonged use of a combined oral contraceptive pill.
T 285. It causes more deaths than any other female genital-tract cancer.

Regarding prophylaxis against venous thromboembolism in women undergoing gynaecological surgery,

T 286. there is increased risk of wound haematoma if heparin is administered near to the site of an abdominal incision.

T 287. platelet counts should be monitored in patients receiving heparin for more than five days.

F 288. in women undergoing radical pelvic surgery, dextran 70 infusion has been shown to reduce the risk of deep-vein thrombosis to approximately 5%.

T 289. heparin enhances anti-thrombin III activity.

There is an increased incidence of postoperative 'burst abdomen' in association with

F 290. mass closure techniques.

T 291. the use of catgut to suture the rectus sheath.

F 292. nonclosure of the parietal peritoneum.

The following statements concerning intestinal obstruction are correct:

T 293. Abdominal distension occurs more often in association with mechanical obstruction than with paralytic ileus.

T 294. Paralytic ileus has a recognised association with hypokalaemia.

The following statements relating to abdominal hysterectomy are correct:

T 295. The operation carries less risk to the bowel than does laparoscopy.

F 296. Prophylactic antibiotic therapy reduces the incidence of vault haematoma.

Regarding endometrial ablation/resection,

F 297. the risk of fluid overload is avoided by the use of less than five litres of irrigant.

F 298. Patients rendered amenorrhoeic following the procedure do not need contraception.

T 299. About 50% of all hysterectomies will be avoided.

T 300. A small proportion of patients will develop cyclical pain.

March 1999

Concerning vaginal ultrasound imaging in early pregnancy,

T 1. absence of cardiac activity in an embryo of 3 cm reliably indicates a non-viable pregnancy.

F 2. an intrauterine gestational sac is reliably seen 20 days from ovulation.

Concerning ultrasound in pregnancy,

F 3. ultrasound markers may be detected during a second-trimester scan in 70% of fetuses with Down syndrome.

T 4. trisomy 18 is the chromosome abnormality most commonly associated with choroid plexus cysts.

T 5. most fetuses with a nuchal translucency of 2.5 mm or more are normal.

The following conditions can be detected by ultrasound screening of the fetus:

T 6. syndactyly.

F 7. Edward syndrome.

T 8. congenital heart block.

With regard to fetal lumbar meningomyelocele,

F 9. the extent of neuromuscular disability can be predicted antenatally.

F 10. there is a recognised association with renal anomalies.

The following conditions are characteristically associated with oligohydramnios:

F 11. fetal imperforate anus.

T 12. talipes equinovarus.

The following conditions would be expected to conform to the pattern of inheritance shown in Figure 3:

F 13. Huntington's chorea.
T 14. Phenylketonuria.
T 15. Tay Sachs disease.

Recognised causes of vomiting in the second trimester of pregnancy include

T 16. necrobiosis in a fibroid.
T 17. trophoblastic disease.

The following statements regarding multiple sclerosis in pregnancy are correct:

T 18. Epidural anaesthesia will not precipitate a relapse.
F 19. The second stage of labour should be shortened.
T 20. It has no effect on the long-term prognosis of the disease.

The following have a recognised association:

F 21. prolonged maternal intravenous infusion : neonatal hyponatraemia.
F 22. epidural analgesia : reduction of fetal heart rate variability.
F 23. migraine : pregnancy-induced hypertension.

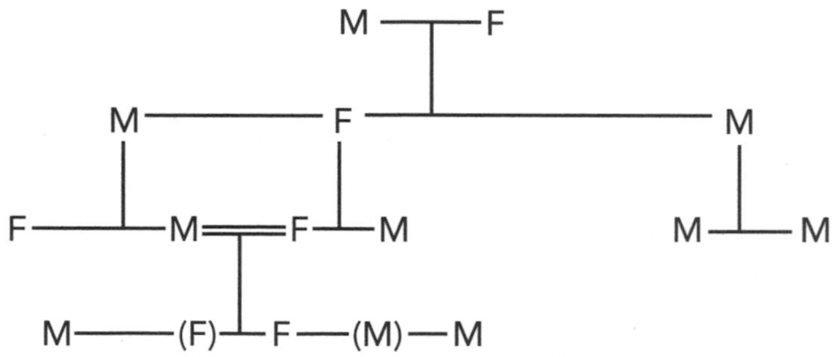

===== : Consanguineous mating

[M = normal male, (M) = affected male, F = normal female, (F) = affected female]

Figure 3

In maternal thyrotoxicosis complicating pregnancy or the puerperium,

F 24. neonatal hyperthyroidism does not occur if the mother has been euthyroid.

T 25. subtotal thyroidectomy is acceptable treatment in the second trimester.

F 26. an increase in the size of the thyroid indicates inadequate treatment.

The following occur more frequently in the pregnant than in the nonpregnant woman:

T 27. erythema nodosum.

F 28. duodenal ulcer.

Impaired glucose tolerance (gestational diabetes) diagnosed for the first time during pregnancy is characteristically associated with

T 29. an increased risk of the subsequent development of diabetes mellitus in later life.

F 30. a need for treatment with insulin in the majority of cases.

F 31. an increased incidence of fetal malformation, even when treated.

The following conditions have an increased incidence in pregnancy complicated by poorly controlled diabetes mellitus:

T 32. fetal oesophageal atresia.

T 33. acute pyelonephritis.

T 34. preterm labour.

Sickle cell anaemia in pregnant women is associated with an increased incidence of

T 35. intrauterine growth retardation.

T 36. megaloblastic anaemia.

A rhesus negative woman with rhesus D antibodies is in the 18th week of her fifth pregnancy. Her last child had haemolytic disease of the newborn and required four postnatal exchange transfusions. This pregnancy is by a different consort whose rhesus genotype is cde/CDD. It therefore follows that

F 37. a positive indirect Coombs test performed on cord blood indicates a child affected by haemolytic disease.

T 38. if an affected fetus requires an intrauterine transfusion then group O rhesus negative blood should be crossmatched against the mother's serum.

F 39. the infant has a 75% chance of being affected with haemolytic disease.

A healthy normotensive woman aged 40 years is pregnant for the first time. Compared with an otherwise similar 25-year-old woman,

T 40. it is significantly more likely that she will have a higher fasting blood glucose concentration.

T 41. she has almost double the likelihood of a twin pregnancy.

F 42. the risk of her baby having a neural tube defect is increased by 10%.

F 43. there is an increased risk of premature rupture of the membranes.

There is a recognised association between intrauterine death of the fetus and

T 44. well-controlled maternal diabetes mellitus.

F 45. herpes simplex virus infection.

T 46. renal agenesis.

The following drugs administered during pregnancy are correctly paired with a recognised unwanted side effect:

T 47. carbimazole : fetal goitre.

F 48. nifedipine : fetal tachycardia.

F 49. 1-thyroxine : neonatal thyrotoxicosis.

In the evaluation of abdominal pain at 24 weeks of pregnancy,

T 50. acute pyelonephritis is more likely on the right than on the left side.

F 51. quiescent ulcerative colitis is liable to relapse during pregnancy.

F 52. an ultrasound scan can exclude a placental abruption.

A 30-year-old woman who has had four previous normal pregnancies and deliveries is admitted to hospital at 30 weeks of gestation. For the past four hours she has had severe generalised abdominal pain. On examination, she is pale and anxious. Her blood pressure is 110/70 mmHg and her pulse rate is 100 beats/minute. The fundal height is 32 cm above the symphysis pubis. The lie is longitudinal but the presentation is difficult to determine because of marked abdominal tenderness. The fetal heart is not audible and no trace is obtained on cardiotocography. The haemoglobin is

10 g/dl, the platelet count is 25,000/mm³, and the fibrin degradation product levels are raised. Oozing from the site of the venepuncture is noted. The following statements are correct:

T 53. Epidural analgesia is contraindicated.
T 54. Depletion of factor VIII is likely.
F 55. Central venous pressure monitoring is indicated.
F 56. The most likely diagnosis is ruptured uterus.

The following statements concerning rubella and pregnancy are correct:

F 57. Maternal infection occurring in the second trimester is followed by the neonatal rubella syndrome in less than 1% of cases.
F 58. Treatment with immunoglobulin reduces the risk of congenital abnormality.
F 59. Rubella vaccination is associated with the neonatal rubella syndrome.

Listeria monocytogenes

F 60. is carried in the intestinal tract of about 20% of the adult UK population.
T 61. multiplies at temperatures as low as 6°C.
F 62. is spread through droplets in the air.

The following maternal symptoms have a recognised association with parvovirus infection:

T 63. polyarthropathy.
T 64. transient aplastic anaemia in those with sickle cell anaemia.

Regarding fetal infection with toxoplasmosis,

F 65. the fetus is more severely affected when infection occurs late in pregnancy.
T 66. when primary infection occurs in pregnancy, the fetus is infected in approximately 40% of cases.
F 67. pregnancy reactivates latent disease.

Clinical manifestations of neonatal cytomegalovirus infection include:

T 68. petechiae.
T 69. cataracts.

The following anti-infective agents are contraindicated in the third trimester of pregnancy:

T 70. chloramphenicol.
F 71. gentamycin sulphate.
F 72. acyclovir.

In a paper describing the use of a new drug for the treatment of hypertension in pregnancy you read: 'The mean fall in diastolic blood pressure in the treated group (n = 30) was 10 mmHg ± 3.0 (SD) and in a control group given placebo (n = 29) the mean fall was 4 mmHg ± 2.6 (SD). Using the t test, P < 0.001'. Assuming a normal distribution, the following statements are correct:

F 73. The most appropriate way to allocate patients to the drug or the placebo group would have been to give the drug or placebo to alternate patients.
F 74. If the trial were properly conducted, the doctors involved should know which patients received the active drug and which the placebo.
T 75. A non-parametric statistical method would also have been valid.

In the long term treatment of hypertension in pregnancy,

T 76. beta-adrenergic drugs impair maternal carbohydrate metabolism.
T 77. hydralazine hydrochloride is an unsuitable drug.

A 23-year-old primigravida with no significant medical history is found to have proteinuria (++) at the booking clinic at 16 weeks. This finding is confirmed on examination of a midstream specimen of urine, which is sterile. Proteinuria persists. The following antenatal investigations are indicated:

T 78. a 24-hour urine protein estimation.
F 79. intravenous urography (pyelography).
T 80. estimation of serum creatinine concentration.

Recognised associations of eclampsia include

T 81. renal cortical necrosis.
F 82. subdural haematoma.

External cephalic version for a singleton breech presentation

T 83. carried out after 36 weeks of gestation significantly reduces the incidence of breech presentation at term.

F 84. is strongly contraindicated when there has been antepartum haemorrhage of any cause.

T 85. should be preceded by an ultrasound scan.

The following conditions have a recognised association with spontaneous preterm labour:

T 86. fetal oesophageal atresia.

F 87. maternal hypertension.

T 88. pregnancy occurring under 16 years of age.

With respect to multiple pregnancy,

T 89. the frequency of monozygotic twins is approximately uniform throughout the world.

F 90. the presence of two separate placentas is diagnostic of dizygotic twins.

When the gestational age is 42 weeks or more,

F 91. there is a substantial fall in the fetal haemoglobin level.

F 92. the most common cause of perinatal death is trauma.

T 93. oligohydramnios is a recognised feature.

Intravaginal prostaglandin E_2 is significantly associated with

F 94. neonatal hyponatraemia.

F 95. neonatal bronchospasm.

Recognised causes of persistent occipitoposterior position of the fetal head include

T 96. uterine fibroids.

F 97. congenital uterine abnormalities.

T 98. an anthropoid pelvis.

F 99. oligohydramnios.

With regard to face presentation at term,

T 100. vaginal delivery is commonly safely achieved with mentoanterior presentation.

F 101. the incidence is increased by the use of epidural analgesia.

F 102. the recorded incidence is approximately 1/150 deliveries.

In labour, following one caesarean section,

F 103. the incidence of rupture of a 'classical' scar is approximately 20%.
T 104. fetal heart rate abnormalities indicate the possibility of scar dehiscence.

There is an increased incidence of prolapse of the umbilical cord with

F 105. postmaturity.
T 106. premature labour.
T 107. the use of Kielland forceps.

Fetal acidosis in labour is characteristically associated with

T 108. prolonged pregnancy.
T 109. fetal intraventricular haemorrhage.
T 110. decreased baseline variability on a cardiotocographic trace.

The following statements concerning continuous lumbar epidural analgesia are correct:

F 111. The procedure must be abandoned if a spinal tap occurs during its administration.
F 112. It is contraindicated where intrauterine growth restriction is suspected.
T 113. Respiratory arrest is a recognised complication.
F 114. It increases the risk of postpartum haemorrhage.

Acute inversion of the uterus may be associated with active management of the third stage of labour and

T 115. the uterus should be replaced immediately whether or not the placenta has separated.
F 116. is a consequence of waiting overlong for the uterus to contract.

In the management of hypovolaemic shock,

F 117. there is negligible risk of acute respiratory distress syndrome (shock lung) unless more than five litres of crystalloid have been transfused.
F 118. there is no danger of pulmonary oedema while the central venous pressure is normal.
T 119. acute renal tubular necrosis is a recognised complication.

Features of disseminated intravascular coagulation include

F 120. an association with systemic lupus erythematosus.
T 121. activation of factor VII.
T 122. the appearance of free plasmin in the circulation.
F 123. reversal of the process by transfusion of stored whole blood.

Recognised associations of major pulmonary thromboembolism include

F 124. a prolonged clotting time.
T 125. protein C deficiency.
F 126. early change in the chest X-ray.
T 127. an inverted T wave on electrocardiogram.

According to the FIGO (international) definition, the calculation of the maternal mortality rate

T 128. excludes those due to fortuitous diseases, for example, carcinoma of the stomach.
F 129. includes only those that occur during pregnancy.
T 130. includes undelivered as well as delivered patients.

Breastfeeding and 'rooming in' (whereby the baby's cot is next to the mother's bed)

T 131. means that the infant is more likely to colonise bacteria from its own mother than from elsewhere.
T 132. reduces the future incidence of 'non-accidental injury'.
F 133. encourages four-hour feeding regimens.
T 134. improves contraction and involution of the uterus.

Drugs considered to be unsuitable for administration to the breastfeeding mother include

F 135. rifampicin.
T 136. senna.
T 137. combined oral contraceptive pill.
T 138. tetracycline.

The following statements concerning puerperal mastitis are correct:

F 139. Suckling should be discouraged on the affected breast.
F 140. Group A streptococci are the commonest causal organisms.
T 141. Penicillinase-resistant antibiotics should be used.

Perinatal mortality rates (PMR) per 1000 births by birth weight are given for two towns X and Y (actual numbers of deaths are given in parenthesis).

Birth weight (g)	TOWN X	TOWN Y
< 1501	317.0 (n = 44)	444.0 (n = 8)
1501–2500	43.7 (n = 36)	60.4 (n = 9)
> 2500	2.54 (n = 35)	2.54 (n = 10)

The following statements, which refer to the above data, are correct:

T 142. It is not possible from the data shown to calculate the overall perinatal mortality rate for town X.

T 143. The difference in mortality for babies < 1501 g in the two towns can be tested by the chi-square test.

F 144. Low birth weight (< 2500 g) accounted for about one in three perinatal deaths.

F 145. More babies (live and stillborn) were delivered in town Y than in town X.

The following statements concerning meconium aspiration are correct:

T 146. It is a recognised feature of post-term pregnancies.

T 147. It can occur prior to labour.

F 148. It is more common following breech delivery.

F 149. It is a common feature of preterm delivery.

Recognised causes of ambiguous genitalia at birth include

F 150. the androgen insensitivity syndrome.

F 151. Klinefelter syndrome.

T 152. severe hypospadias.

Septic abortion/miscarriage, when associated with a *Clostridium perfringens* (*welchii*) infection, has the following recognised features:

T 153. haemolysis.

T 154. hypotension.

T 155. acute respiratory distress syndrome.

In women with choriocarcinoma,

F 156. a rise in the level of urinary human chorionic gonadotrophin, after initial clinical response, is diagnostic of recurrence.
T 157. if relapse occurs, it is most commonly within one year of treatment.
F 158. there is usually a recent history of first-trimester miscarriage.

Recognised features of Turner syndrome include

F 159. a mosaic pattern (45X0/46XX) in approximately 50% of cases.
F 160. absence of withdrawal bleeding after treatment with hormone therapy.

An individual of female phenotype with gonadal dysgenesis and an XY karyotype characteristically

T 161. has a vagina.
F 162. has galactorrhoea.

Regarding precocious puberty,

T 163. breast development precedes the onset of menstruation.
T 164. it is usually idiopathic.
T 165. when idiopathic, it may be treated with cyproterone acetate.

The following statements regarding normal puberty are correct:

T 166. Anovulatory cycles are common in the first 12 months after the menarche.
F 167. The maximal growth spurt occurs after the menarche.

A 17-year-old girl with no secondary sex characteristics is currently studying for university entrance. She has never menstruated. She is 1.60 m (5 ft 3 in) tall, weighs 47.6 kg (7 st 7 lb) and has a body mass index of 18.6. Laboratory results are reported as: karyotype XX; plasma follicle-stimulating hormone 5.0 iu/l; plasma luteinising hormone 6.2 iu/l and plasma prolactin 300 mu/l. The following statements are correct:

F 168. A probable diagnosis is androgen insensitivity.
F 169. X-ray of the skull is mandatory.
F 170. Laparoscopy is necessary to establish the cause.

Premature ovarian failure

T 171. is a recognised complication of mumps.
F 172. is a characteristic feature of anorexia nervosa.
T 173. predisposes to the development of coronary artery disease.
F 174. is associated with the absence of primordial follicles.

In women with objectively measured idiopathic heavy menstrual bleeding,

T 175. more than 90% are ovulating normally.
F 176. curettage is of therapeutic benefit.

The following symptoms are correctly paired with a recognised cause:

F 177. hirsutism : prolactinoma.
F 178. diplopia : avascular necrosis of the pituitary.
T 179. intermenstrual bleeding : chlamydial endometritis.

The combination of inappropriate lactation and secondary amenorrhoea is a recognised association of

F 180. hyperthyroidism.
T 181. acromegaly.

Recognised associations of polycystic ovary syndrome include

F 182. spasmodic dysmenorrhoea.
F 183. carcinoma of the breast.
T 184. carcinoma of the endometrium.

Prolactin secretion is inhibited by

F 185. ethinyloestradiol.
F 186. lithium carbonate.
T 187. cabergoline.

An 18-year-old woman presents with right iliac fossa pain and a heavy vaginal discharge. Her last menstrual period was six weeks earlier. She had been regularly taking a combined oral contraceptive for the past eight months. She is apyrexial. Abdominal examination reveals a poorly localised area of tenderness in the right iliac fossa. Vaginal examination shows no abnormality. Results of investigation include: urine microscopy –

numerous pus cells; haemoglobin 9 g/dl; white-cell count 10⁹l. The following courses of action are appropriate:

F 188. Perform a plain X-ray of the abdomen.
F 189. Arrange urgent laparoscopy.
F 190. Prescribe antibiotics.

The incidence of vaginal candidiasis is increased

F 191. in postmenopausal women.
T 192. in women with ulcerative colitis.

Procedures of value in the diagnosis of acute gonorrhoea in the female include

F 193. culture of a high vaginal swab.
T 194. urethral swabs from her sexual partner.

Bacterial vaginosis

F 195. can be diagnosed on culture of a high vaginal swab.
T 196. is associated with an increased number of anaerobes.
T 197. can be successfully treated with intravaginal clindamycin.

The following statements concerning the human immunodeficiency virus (HIV1) are correct:

F 198. Sexual transmission is reduced by the use of spermicides.
T 199. The spread of infection to healthcare attendants is lessened by the measures which are effective against the spread of hepatitis B.

Contraindications to the use of the intrauterine contraceptive device include

F 200. woman's age over 40 years.
F 201. previous cone biopsy.

Following the insertion of an intrauterine contraceptive device,

F 202. the expulsion rate after the first year is at least 20%.
F 203. a typical pregnancy rate after the first year is 4/100 woman years.

The following metabolic changes occur with the use of the combined oral contraceptive pill:

F 204. there is a decrease in plasma pyridoxine concentrations.
T 205. endogenous progesterone concentrations fall.
T 206. serum ferritin concentrations rise.

The following statements about methods of contraception are correct:

T 207. Oil-based creams and gels adversely affect the efficacy of the male condom.
F 208. Most diaphragms are impregnated with nonoxynol-9.

With laparoscopic clip sterilisation

F 209. there is a failure rate of approximately 0.2%.
F 210. most deaths are due to anaesthetic complications.
F 211. the procedure should not be performed during menstruation.

The following conditions are correctly paired with a recognised cause:

T 212. reversible oligozoospermia : sulfasalazine.
T 213. asthenospermia : Kartagener syndrome.
T 214. impotence : hyperprolactinaemia.

Clomifene citrate is a recognised treatment for

F 215. primary amenorrhoea.
F 216. premature menopause.
F 217. galactorrhoea.

Assisted conception using ovum donation should be considered in women with

T 218. repeated poor response to gonadotrophin stimulation.
T 219. resistant ovarian syndrome.
F 220. Asherman syndrome.
F 221. androgen insensitivity.

With regard to endometriosis,

T 222. medroxyprogesterone acetate is a recommended drug in the treatment of symptomatic mild to moderate disease.

T 223. it is more common in women with müllerian duct abnormalities.
F 224. local lymphocyte beta-cell activity is increased.

Recognised complications of pelvic endometriosis include

F 225. anovulatory cycles.
F 226. vaginal adenosis.
F 227. postmenopausal bleeding.

Recognised side effects of the administration of danazol include

T 228. arthralgia.
T 229. dryness of the vagina.
F 230. galactorrhoea.

Gonadotrophin-releasing hormone (GnRH) analogue administration

F 231. should be discontinued if ovarian hyperstimulation occurs.
T 232. induces ovulation in patients with hypogonadotrophic amenorrhoea.
F 233. is associated with an increased incidence of acne vulgaris.

Recognised causes of postmenopausal bleeding include

F 234. preinvasive carcinoma of the cervix.
T 235. prolapsed urethral mucosa.
F 236. subserous fibroids.
F 237. hepatic cirrhosis.

A 60-year-old married woman presents with a history of recent vaginal bleeding. On examination, the cervix appears healthy, the uterus is small and atrophic and no abnormality is felt in the adnexa. A cervical smear is reported as showing cells suspicious of malignancy, possibly columnar. In the management of this patient

F 238. the smear should be repeated prior to further investigation.
F 239. cone biopsy is appropriate treatment.
F 240. adenocarcinoma of the endocervix is the most likely diagnosis.

A postmenopausal woman exhibits the following changes:

T 241. atrophic trigonitis of the bladder.
F 242. a reduction in the serum cholesterol concentration.

Oestrogen replacement therapy is of value in

F 243. lichen sclerosus.
F 244. nocturnal frequency of micturition.

Frequency of micturition is a recognised feature of

T 245. trichomonal vaginitis.
T 246. papilloma of the bladder.
F 247. vesicovaginal fistula.

Urodynamic studies

F 248. can distinguish between neuropathic and idiopathic detrusor overactivity.
T 249. measure the variation in 'detrusor' pressure during bladder filling.
F 250. necessitate the use of video equipment.

The aims of surgery for the relief of stress incontinence of urine include

F 251. reduction of the functional length of the urethra.
T 252. correction of funnelling at the bladder neck.
T 253. an increase in urethral resistance.

The following may lead to genital prolapse in parous women:

T 254. pudendal nerve damage.
F 255. breastfeeding.

Genital prolapse is best treated non-surgically

F 256. in a patient with recurrent prolapse after vaginal hysterectomy and repair.
T 257. in a patient who wishes to have a subsequent vaginal delivery.

The following are correctly paired:

F 258. severe vulvovaginitis : group A haemolytic streptococcal infection.
T 259. recurrent ulceration of the labia minora : Behcet's disease.
T 260. vaginal petechiae :aplastic anaemia.

The vulval skin

F 261. contains cellular atypia in more than 25% of cases of hypertrophic dystrophy.

T   262.   is involved in trichomonal infection.

T   263.   is a site for psoriasis.

In primary carcinoma of the fallopian tube,

F   264.   the tumour is bilateral in approximately 60% of cases.

F   265.   transcoelomic spread rarely occurs.

F   266.   radiotherapy is the treatment of choice.

T   267.   a profuse watery vaginal discharge is a characteristic symptom.

Cervical ectopy

F   268.   is more common in progestogen-only oral contraceptive users than in users of intrauterine contraceptive devices.

F   269.   has the histological features of an ulcer.

A 25-year-old parous woman whose cervical smear showed moderate and then severe dyskaryosis has a colposcopic examination that shows no abnormality. The following treatments are appropriate:

F   270.   knife conisation.

T   271.   a repeat smear in three months time.

F   272.   laser vaporisation.

A 45-year-old woman is found to have a friable tumour on the anterior lip of the cervix with extension to the left parametrium. Histology of the tumour is squamous-cell carcinoma. An intravenous urogram (IVU) shows left hydroureter and left hydronephrosis. Cystoscopy reveals bullous oedema. The following statements are correct:

F   273.   A diagnosis of stage IV carcinoma of the cervix can be made with confidence.

T   274.   The patient's blood urea is likely to be normal.

In stage IIb carcinoma of the cervix

T   275.   radiotherapy is the treatment of choice.

F   276.   colposcopy is indicated before treatment.

With regard to adenocarcinoma of the uterus,

T   277.   in stage I disease, the incidence of pelvic lymph node metastasis is approximately 3%.

F 278. the removal of a vaginal cuff at the time of hysterectomy for stage I disease reduces the incidence of vault recurrence.
F 279. preoperative treatment with progestogens improves the prognosis.

Endometrial carcinoma

F 280. metastasises characteristically to the supraclavicular lymph nodes.
F 281. is a sequel to prenatal oestrogen therapy.

With regard to serum tumour markers in ovarian malignancy,

F 282. a raised serum CA125 (carcinoma antigen) concentration is found in association with approximately 40% of epithelial tumours.
F 283. alphafetoprotein (AFP) concentration may be raised in association with a dysgerminoma.
F 284. carcino-embryonic antigen (CEA) concentration is more commonly raised in association with serous than with mucinous tumours.

Five-year survival in stage III ovarian cancer is improved by

F 285. adjuvant pelvic radiotherapy.
F 286. para-aortic lymphadenectomy.
F 287. intraperitoneal alkylating agents.

The following have a recognised association:

T 288. Crohn's disease : right hydronephrosis.
T 289. diverticular disease : vaginal fistula formation.
F 290. colorectal carcinoma : vegetarianism.

Cryosurgery is recognised as effective in the treatment of

F 291. vulval intraepithelial neoplasia (VIN).
F 292. cervical intraepithelial neoplasia stage 3 (CIN3).
T 293. discrete condylomata accuminata.

For the first 18 hours after a difficult abdominal hysterectomy a patient fails to void urine. The following statements are correct:

F 294. The most likely cause is prolonged hypovolaemia.
T 295. If due to ureteric injury, she should be treated by nephrostomies and definitive ureteric repair three months later.
F 296. She is best managed by dialysis until the diagnosis is established.

The following are recognised causes of a delay of more than 30 minutes in the recovery after general anaesthesia:

T 297. severe hypoxia during anaesthesia.
T 298. hypothyroidism.
T 299. concurrent use of hypotensive drugs.

September 1999

Nuchal translucency

F 1. is diagnostic of a chromosomal abnormality.

The following features observed on antenatal ultrasound scanning are associated with Turner syndrome:

T 2. hydrops fetalis at 20 weeks of gestation.
T 3. structural heart anomalies.

Ultrasonic features of intrauterine growth retardation include

F 4. an increased incidence of fetal breathing movements.
T 5. maximum amniotic pool depth less than 2 cm.
T 6. increased pulsatility index in the umbilical arteries.

Chorionic villus sampling (CVS)

T 7. may diagnose a chromosome abnormality not expressed in the fetus.
T 8. increases the risk of limb reduction deformities.
T 9. is associated with a higher false positive rate than is amniocentesis.

Fetal blood sampling during the antenatal period

F 10. is necessary for the diagnosis of fetal beta-thalassaemia.
F 11. results in 10–15% incidence of premature rupture of the membranes.
T 12. is indicated in the investigation of fetal hydrops.

Examination of the amniotic fluid allows a specific diagnosis of

T 13. Hurler's syndrome.
F 14. fetal exomphalos.
T 15. retinoblastoma.

The following conditions would be expected to conform to the pattern of inheritance shown in Figure 4:

F 16. glucose-6-phosphate dehydrogenase deficiency.
T 17. Huntington's chorea.
T 18. osteogenesis imperfecta.

The following disorders are correctly associated with the mode of inheritance:

T 19. Duchenne's disease (hypertrophic muscular dystrophy) : X-linked recessive.
T 20. Tay-Sach's disease : autosomal recessive.

With regard to Down syndrome,

F 21. if the mother is a carrier of balanced translocation (type 21/13–15) the risk of a child being born with Down syndrome is 50%.
F 22. the incidence in babies born to women over 40 years is between 5% and 10%.
T 23. 95% are of the non-dysjunctional variety.
F 24. the paternal chromosome constitution is irrelevant.

Achondroplasia

F 25. is the most common lethal chondrodystrophy.
F 26. can be excluded by a normal fetal femur length measured by ultrasound at 18 weeks of pregnancy.

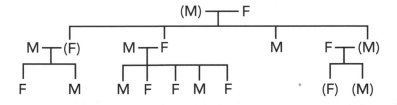

[M = normal male, (M) = affected male, F = normal female, (F) = affected female]

Figure 4

Congenital toxoplasmosis is associated with

T   27.   hydrocephalus.

F   28.   hepatitis.

Consumption of the following is associated with human listerial infection:

F   29.   tinned corned beef.

T   30.   coleslaw.

F   31.   freshly roasted shoulder of lamb.

Congenital infection with cytomegalovirus

T   32.   is associated with intracerebral calcification.

T   33.   can be detected by culture of the infant's urine.

The following statements relating to vaccination are correct:

F   34.   If vaccination against poliomyelitis is required in pregnancy, the Sabin strain should be employed.

F   35.   human varicella zoster immunoglobulin should be given to the term newborn of a mother who has had chickenpox during the second trimester.

F   36.   Rubella vaccination in early pregnancy is an indication for termination.

Intrahepatic cholestasis in pregnancy is characteristically associated with

T   37.   elevated total bile acids in the blood.

F   38.   elevated serum concentrations of the direct bilirubin fraction.

The following conditions and features occurring in pregnancy are appropriately paired:

F   39.   hyperthyroidism : acne.

T   40.   systemic lupus erythematosus : thrombocytopenia.

There is an increased incidence of deep vein thrombosis in pregnant women

T   41.   who are aged over 40 years.

F   42.   who deliver precipitously.

The following statements regarding thyrotoxicosis complicating pregnancy and the puerperium are correct:

T 43. Neonatal goitre is a recognised complication of overtreatment.
F 44. Neonatal thyrotoxicosis is clinically apparent within 24 hours of birth.
F 45. Breastfeeding is contraindicated if a mother is taking propylthiouracil.

Regarding systemic lupus erythematosus in pregnancy,

F 46. azathioprine therapy should be discontinued because of adverse effect on the fetus.
T 47. exacerbations of maternal disease occur commonly in the puerperium.
F 48. fetal heart block occurs in at least 40% of babies.

Patients with acute pyelonephritis in pregnancy

F 49. have an increased likelihood of a malformation of the urogenital tract.
F 50. should have a cystoscopy after the pregnancy.

Recognised features of sickle cell disease complicating pregnancy include

T 51. an increased incidence of spontaneous miscarriage.
F 52. an increased incidence of iron deficiency.
F 53. reduced sensitivity to oxytocics.
T 54. an increased incidence of severe pregnancy-induced hypertension.

Thalassaemia major is

T 55. a microcytic hypochromic variety of anaemia.
F 56. caused by heterozygous inheritance of thalassaemia genes.
T 57. associated with secondary amenorrhoea.

In patients with gestational diabetes

T 58. there is a history of parental diabetes mellitus in about 25% of cases.
F 59. less than 2% will develop impaired glucose tolerance within five years.

In pregnancy complicated by diabetes mellitus, the following have a recognised association:

T 60.   a sharp increase in insulin requirements : intrauterine death in the last four weeks.

F 61.   mild recurrent hypoglycaemia : an increased risk of fetal abnormality.

T 62.   persistently high $HbA1_c$: an increased risk of fetal abnormality.

In pregnancy complicated by insulin-dependent diabetes mellitus

F 63.   insulin requirements tend to rise immediately after the birth.

T 64.   the incidence of pregnancy-induced hypertension is increased.

Maternal pulmonary oedema following use of beta-agonist tocolytic agents is associated with

T 65.   the use of intravenous saline.

Complications arising during the administration of ritodrine are more likely when there is

T 66.   maternal anaemia of less than 9 g/dl.

T 67.   concomitant use of steroids.

F 68.   dehydration.

T 69.   maternal diabetes.

An increased intake of folic acid is required when pregnancy is associated with

F 70.   the administration of ampicillin.

T 71.   sickle cell disease.

T 72.   malaria.

F 73.   asymptomatic bacteriuria.

In patients undergoing anticoagulation with warfarin sodium

F 74.   the effects of the drug are antagonised within ten minutes by intravenous administration of vitamin K.

F 75.   breastfeeding is contraindicated.

Cigarette smoking in pregnancy is associated with

F 76.   pregnancy-induced hypertension.

F 77.   neonatal thrombocytopenia.

Intramuscular pethidine in labour

F 78.   is eliminated from the neonate within 24 hours of delivery.
F 79.   produces maximal neonatal respiratory depression if given within the hour before delivery.
T 80.   slows maternal gastric emptying.

In a pregnant woman over the age of 35 years, there is a recognised increase in the

F 81.   incidence of pregnancy prolonged beyond 40 weeks of gestation.
F 82.   frequency of fetal neural tube defects.

Placental abruption

F 83.   occurs in approximately 10% of otherwise uncomplicated pregnancies.
F 84.   causes postpartum haemorrhage only when hypofibrinogenaemia develops.
F 85.   is associated with antecedent hypertension in about 80% of cases.

A recognised association exists between polyhydramnios and

F 86.   congenital fetal adrenal hyperplasia.
F 87.   fetal polycystic kidneys.

Reduction in uteroplacental blood flow has a recognised association with

T 88.   the second stage of labour.
T 89.   neonatal polycythaemia.

Chorioamnionitis

F 90.   can usually be prevented by the use of prophylactic antibiotics.

The following statements, which refer to the data in the table overleaf, are correct:

F 91.   In the study described, patients were allocated alternately to 'rested' and 'ambulant' groups.
T 92.   The value of '$P = 0.022$' suggests that the observed difference did not occur by chance.
T 93.   The value of 't' refers to a test for the difference between the means.
F 94.   Among the 'ambulant', 95% of oestriol values were between 365.6 ± 197.1.

Forty pregnant patients participated in a randomised controlled trial of complete bed rest versus ambulation in the management of proteinuric hypertension. The measurement of urinary oestriol (nmol/litre) in the two groups was as follows:

	Rested group (n = 20)	Ambulant group (n = 20)
Mean	209.9	365.6
Standard deviation	70.3	197.1
Range	180–1200	115–860

t = 2.08, difference between means = 155.7, P = 0.022

The following statements concerning eclampsia are correct:

T 95. Antepartum eclampsia has a higher maternal mortality rate than has intrapartum eclampsia.

F 96. The fit occurs following delivery in less than 10% of cases.

Amniotic fluid embolism is characteristically associated with

T 97. prolonged labour.

T 98. infusion of oxytocin.

The following lesion is correctly paired with a recognised clinical association:

T 99. postpartum haemorrhage : maternal renal cortical necrosis.

F 100. placental chorioangioma : oligohydramnios.

With regard to lower-segment caesarean section

T 101. the subsequent vaginal delivery rate in those allowed to labour is greater than 65%.

T 102. an associated general anaesthetic is the main cause of maternal death.

Concerning shoulder dystocia,

T 103. brachial plexus injury involves cervical nerve roots 5 and 6 more frequently than 7 and 8.

T 104. for a given birth weight it occurs more often in babies of diabetic mothers.

T 105. in babies weighing more than 5 kg at birth delivered vaginally the incidence is approximately 50%.

Recognised causes of prolongation of the first stage of labour include

106. epidural analgesia.
107. maternal keto-acidosis.

With regard to the management of breech presentation at term,

108. cord prolapse occurs in 5% of cases with footling presentation.
109. pelvimetry should be performed before consideration of vaginal delivery.

Recognised associations exist between a transverse lie of the fetus in a multiparous patient at 38 weeks of gestation and

110. fetal renal agenesis.
111. excessive fetal extensor muscle tone.

Epidural analgesia

112. should not be commenced during the second stage of labour.

Factors predisposing to maternal pulmonary aspiration of gastric contents during labour include

113. the administration of an oxytocic for the third stage.

With regard to preterm breech,

114. meta-analysis of randomised controlled trials has shown that caesarean section is the optimal mode of delivery.
115. regardless of the mode of delivery, neonatal mortality and morbidity are higher at any given gestation than with cephalic presentation.

Intravenous oxytocin is indicated for the management of the third stage with

116. a previous history of postpartum haemorrhage.
117. hypertrophic obstructive cardiomyopathy.

The following statements about breastfeeding are correct:

118. The risk of transmission of HIV through breast milk is highest for babies whose mothers seroconvert after delivery.

F   119. It should be discontinued if the mother suffers a cracked nipple.

The following are recognised to be of proven benefit:

F   120. immunotherapy with paternal leucocytes to prevent recurrent miscarriage.

T   121. external cephalic version after 36 completed weeks of pregnancy.

T   122. induction of labour after 41 weeks, using prostaglandins if appropriate.

F   123. umbilical arterial Doppler studies in normal pregnancy.

Hydrops fetalis (not due to rhesus isoimmunisation) is a recognised complication of

T   124. fetal thalassaemia.

F   125. fetal renal agenesis.

T   126. cystic adenomatoid malformation of the lung.

T   127. fetal paroxysmal tachycardia.

Recognised associations of persistent patent ductus in the neonate include

T   128. the congenital rubella syndrome.

F   129. the administration of indomethacin prenatally.

A healthy woman of average height and weight had an uncomplicated pregnancy and delivered spontaneously at term. Her blood group is O, rhesus positive, with anti-A activity detected. The baby, a male weighing 2.66 kg, was apparently well at birth but became jaundiced at 48 hours. His direct Coombs test was negative and serum bilirubin concentration 255 micromol/l. Phototherapy was started but despite this his serum bilirubin concentration increased to 357 micromol/l by 60 hours. His haemoglobin concentration was 15 g/dl and his direct Coombs test remained negative, but large numbers of microspherocytes were observed in a film of his peripheral blood. Taking account of this history, the following statements are correct:

T   130   Phototherapy relies on the conversion of unconjugated bilirubin to the conjugated form by the action of ultraviolet light.

F   131. In mothers of blood group O, anti-A and anti-B activity is present in both immunoglobulin M and immunoglobulin G fractions.

T   132. The infant requires exchange transfusion.

Neonatal jaundice appearing on the third day and still present at two weeks of age may be due to

F 133. haemolytic disease of the newborn due to rhesus incompatibility.
T 134. galactosaemia.
T 135. atresia of the bile ducts.

In the preterm baby

T 136. antibiotics are indicated in the presence of features of respiratory distress syndrome.
F 137. the commonest intracranial complication is subarachnoid haemorrhage.
F 138. planned forceps delivery is advised to facilitate any vaginal delivery.

Recognised causes of spontaneous miscarriage include

F 139. an intravenous urogram in early pregnancy.
F 140. systemic corticosteroid therapy in early pregnancy.

Recognised aetiological factors in spontaneous first-trimester miscarriage include

T 141. folate deficiency.
F 142. cervical incompetence.
T 143. coeliac disease.

A non-sensitised rhesus-negative woman undergoes aspiration termination of pregnancy under general anaesthesia at eight weeks of gestation and loses 650 ml of blood. The following statement is correct:

F 144. Haemorrhage of this volume occurs in approximately 10% of terminations performed at this stage of gestation.

The following statements regarding tubal pregnancy are true:

F 145. Evidence of previous tubal infection is present in 75% of cases.
T 146. It accounts for a greater maternal mortality than caesarean section.

Following the evacuation of a non-invasive (complete) hydatidiform mole

F 147. the measurement of 13-subunit hCG is invalidated by the administration of an oral contraceptive.

T 148. approximately 3% of patients develop choriocarcinoma.

Choriocarcinoma

F 149. even with optimal treatment, has a five-year survival rate of less than 70%.

T 150. responds to treatment with folic acid antagonists.

Prenatal stilboestrol administration predisposes to

F 151. precocious breast development in the neonate.

T 152. hypoplasia of the fallopian tubes.

Recognised causes of vaginal bleeding in a girl aged seven years include

T 153. sarcoma botryoides.

T 154. *Enterobius vermicularis* infestation.

Recognised causes of vaginal discharge before the menarche include

T 155. ectopic ureter.

T 156. clear-cell carcinoma of the vagina.

The 47 XXX karyotype

F 157. is characteristically associated with short stature.

T 158. is a recognised cause of premature menopause.

Klinefelter syndrome (47XXY) is characteristically associated with

T 159. impotence.

T 160. a raised serum follicle-stimulating hormone level.

A 16-year-old unmarried girl of Mediterranean origin is referred with primary amenorrhoea. She is 145 cm tall and weighs 47 kg. She has what she regards as an excessive growth of facial hair. Vaginal examination is not possible, as she is virgo intacta with a perforate hymen. Her karyotype is 46XX. In this patient

T 161. an elevated plasma 17-alpha-hydroxyprogesterone concentration is consistent with a diagnosis of congenital adrenal hyperplasia.

F 162. a serum prolactin concentration of 800 mu/l (normal range 200–400 mu/l) confirms a pituitary cause for her amenorrhoea.

Secondary amenorrhoea is a recognised feature of

T 163. anorexia nervosa.

F 164. Down syndrome.

The following are recognised predisposing factors for secondary dysmenorrhoea:

T 165. endometrial resection.

F 166. hyperprolactinaemia.

Regarding hirsutism,

F 167. the severity correlates with the total serum testosterone concentration.

T 168. most affected women have polycystic ovary disease.

The serum concentration of prolactin is

T 169. depressed by levodopa administration.

T 170. increased in polycystic ovary syndrome.

In a 30-year-old woman, serum gonadotrophin concentrations are raised

F 171. following the use of depot progestogen for contraception.

T 172. in the resistant ovary syndrome.

The following disorders are recognised unwanted effects of the drugs with which they are paired:

T 173. hair loss : clomifene citrate.

F 174. hypertension : bromocriptine.

Danazol

T 175. causes a reduction in total thyroxine levels.

Gonadotrophin-releasing hormone (GnRH) agonist analogues

F 176. are the treatment of choice for ovarian endometrioma.

F 177. cause irreversible cortical bone loss within six months of treatment.

GnRH analogues in assisted conception

F 178. reduce the risk of excessive follicle recruitment.

Recognised causes of infertility in the male include

T 179. cystic fibrosis.
T 180. atenolol therapy.

Concerning intrauterine insemination,

T 181. it can legally be performed in the UK without a licence from the Human Fertilisation and Embryology Authority.
F 182. in unexplained infertility, live birth rates of greater than 20% per treatment can be obtained.
T 183. it is an effective treatment for oligozoospermic infertility.

Ovulation stimulation in association with *in vitro* fertilisation

F 184. should be abandoned because of the high risk of hyperstimulation if more than five mature follicles are detected.

Concerning the ovarian hyperstimulation syndrome,

F 185. the severe form affects 2–5% of *in vitro* fertilisation procedures.

The following abnormalities are correctly paired with a recognised cause:

T 186. retrograde ejaculation : diabetic neuropathy.
T 187. oligozoospermia : sulfasalazine therapy.

Predisposing factors among women attending a sexual dysfunction clinic include

T 188. infertility.

Bacterial (anaerobic) vaginosis is associated with

F 189. vaginal erythema.

The following statements regarding the human immunodeficiency virus (HIV) are correct:

F 190. Prevalence rates worldwide are doubling approximately every six months.

F 191. Intravenous drug abusers are the major source of the virus in the UK.

Late sequelae of salpingitis characteristically include

T 192. ectopic pregnancy.
F 193. psoas abscess.

There is a recognised association between Gram negative septicaemia and

T 194. disseminated intravascular coagulation.
T 195. enterocolitis.

In women with objectively measured heavy menstruation

F 196. placebo treatment will reduce the volume of blood lost.
F 197. endometrial hyperplasia can be excluded by ultrasound scanning.

With regard to myomectomy,

F 198. in the event of more than 15 myomata needing to be removed the patient should undergo hysterectomy.

A 30-year-old married woman had an intrauterine contraceptive device fitted five years ago after the birth of her second child. She complains of continuous vaginal bleeding for two months and of recent lower abdominal discomfort. Her lower abdomen appears slightly distended and on vaginal examination the thread of the IUCD is visible, the uterus is of normal size and there is pain on palpation in the Pouch of Douglas. The following statements are correct:

T 199. A positive monoclonal antibody test for 13-subunit human chorionic gonadotrophin would alter the immediate management of the case.
F 200. The patient should be admitted to hospital for immediate laparoscopy.

With regard to female sterilisation

T 201. when failure occurs it is the commonest cause of litigation in gynaecological practice.
F 202. it may be performed in an emergency without the patient's consent.

A nulliparous 25-year-old woman presents with a six-month history of intermittent bilateral lower abdominal pain. She also complains of deep dyspareunia. Laparoscopy shows widespread deposits of endometriosis involving the ovaries and pouch of Douglas and in the utero sacral ligaments. Appropriate treatment options include

T 203. laparotomy and surgical excision of the endometriosis.
F 204. transcervical resection of the endometrium.

Irregular uterine bleeding in a woman aged 45 years is recognised to be associated with

F 205. adenomyosis.
F 206. diabetes mellitus.
T 207. hypothyroidism.

Climacteric (perimenopausal) physiological changes account for

F 208. cervical ectropion.

The following statements regarding hormone replacement therapy (HRT) are correct:

F 209. 90% of women who take long-term unopposed oestrogen therapy develop endometrial hyperplasia.
F 210. Its use significantly increases the incidence of malignant melanoma.

Urethral mucosal prolapse

T 211. is rare before the menopause.
T 212. recurs after surgical treatment.
F 213. is associated with urge incontinence of urine.

Cystocele is a recognised cause of

T 214. genuine stress incontinence.

Three years after vaginal hysterectomy, a 50-year-old woman develops an enterocele. The following operations would be appropriate and would allow preservation of sexual function:

F 215. sacrocolpopexy.
F 216. sacrospinous fixation.
F 217. Burch colposuspension.

Genuine stress incontinence

F 218. does not occur in nulliparous women.

A confused 80-year-old widow is admitted as an emergency. She gives a six-month history of frequency of micturition and recent abdominal distension, constipation and dribbling urinary incontinence. Her temperature is 37.5°C and her blood pressure is 110/70 mmHg. Abdominal examination reveals a soft fluctuant mass arising from the pelvis; there are no other abnormalities on pelvic examination. Urine microscopy reveals significant pyuria and haematuria. Plasma biochemistry is reported as: potassium 4.9 mmol/l; urea 18.4 mmol/l; creatinine 214 micromol/l. The following statements relating to this patient are correct:

F 219. Cystoscopy and urethral dilatation should be undertaken as a matter of urgency.

F 220. In view of the impaired renal function, isotope renography should be performed.

Procedures of value in the investigation of pruritus vulvae include

T 221. examination of the oral cavity.

T 222. biopsy of the vulva.

Recognised associations exist between pruritus ani and

T 223. anal fissure.

F 224. *Ascaris lumbricoides* infestation.

The following statements are correct:

F 225. Fetal exposure to diethylstilboestrol predisposes to squamous-cell carcinoma of the vagina.

F 226. Carcinoma of the fallopian tube is usually of the squamous-cell type.

In malignant disease of the vulva

F 227. carcinoma of Bartholin's gland spreads initially to the internal iliac nodes.

F 228. adenocarcinoma occurs in 25% of cases.

The following statements regarding the management of women with treated cervical intraepithelial neoplasia (CIN) are correct:

F 229. Women who have undergone LLETZ (large loop excision of the transformation zone) are at significantly increased risk of miscarriage.

F 230. Recurrent CIN with glandular changes should be treated by hysterectomy.

The following statements relating to cone biopsy are correct:

T 231. Haematometra is a complication.

F 232. It should only be performed if all the lesion is visible at colposcopy.

In the treatment of invasive carcinoma of the cervix

T 233. proctitis is a recognised complication during therapy.

F 234. surgery is the treatment of choice for stage IIb.

With regard to adenocarcinoma of the cervix,

F 235. subsequent to treatment, oestrogen replacement therapy is contraindicated.

F 236. In stage Ib disease, it carries a worse prognosis than squamous carcinoma.

T 237. It is less radiosensitive than squamous carcinoma.

Doxorubicin hydrochloride (adriamycin)

F 238. is the drug of first choice for treatment of adenocarcinoma of the cervix.

T 239. is cardiotoxic.

Characteristics of atypical endometrial hyperplasia include

T 240. foci of squamous metaplasia.

F 241. premenstrual syndrome.

The incidence of endometrial carcinoma is increased in association with

T 242. a late menopause.

F 243. hypothyroidism.

Endometrial carcinoma

F 244. has a recognised association with previous oral contraceptive therapy.

T 245. has a better prognosis when it occurs below the age of 45 years.

The likelihood of malignancy is increased if an ovarian tumour is associated with

F 246. multiparity.

F 247. torsion.

Features that suggest an ovarian tumour is malignant include

T 248. rapid growth.

T 249. bilateral ovarian involvement.

Elevated serum alphafetoprotein concentrations are tumour markers for

F 250. leiomyosarcoma of the uterus.

F 251. choriocarcinoma of the ovary.

Ovarian dysgerminomas

T 252. are histologically identical to seminomata of the testes.

T 253. are highly radiosensitive.

T 254. most commonly occur in the second and third decades of life.

Primary ovarian adenocarcinoma has a recognised association with

F 255. high parity.

T 256. primary breast cancer.

Cytotoxic therapy is the recommended treatment for

F 257. borderline epithelial tumours of the ovary.

F 258. FIGO stage Ia epithelial carcinoma of the ovary.

The following are recognised features of carcinoma of the female breast:

F 259. systemic spread occurring frequently before the patient appreciates the presence of a tumour.

F 260. bleeding from the nipple at lactation.

The following statements concerning acute abdominal pain are correct:

F 261. Urgent surgical intervention is indicated in patients who present with an appendicular mass.

T 262. A normal white-cell count does not exclude a diagnosis of appendicitis.

A transverse suprapubic incision

F 263. is associated with less haematoma formation than is a midline incision.

F 264. is contraindicated for preterm caesarean section.

Recognised features of postoperative paralytic (adynamic) ileus include

F 265. colicky abdominal pain.

F 266. thirst.

T 267. hypokalaemia.

Twenty-four hours after vaginal hysterectomy, a patient complains of a continuous flow of clear fluid from the vagina. Speculum examination shows it to be coming from the vault wound. Dye passed into the bladder by catheter does not appear in the vagina. The following statements are correct:

F 268. An intravenous urogram is contraindicated.

F 269. Corrective surgery should be performed without delay.

The following statements concerning the management of sudden cardiac arrest are correct:

F 270. Metabolic acidosis occurs within two minutes of the arrest.

March 2000

Congenital anomalies that can be diagnosed by ultrasound imaging at 18 weeks of gestation include

1. Down syndrome.
2. congenital dislocation of the hip.
3. congenital adrenal hyperplasia.
4. phocomelia.

Regarding the fetal heart,

5. The risk of abnormality is 1:10 if a mother has congenital heart disease.

Abnormally high serum concentrations of human chorionic gonadotrophin in pregnancy are associated with

6. fetal erythroblastosis.
7. chorioangioma of the placenta.
8. maternal alcoholism.

Diagnostic amniocentesis at 16 weeks of gestation is associated with an increased incidence of

9. talipes equinovarus.
10. neonatal respiratory difficulty.
11. meconium ileus.

Analysis of a sample of amniotic fluid obtained by amniocentesis assists in the diagnosis of

12. Tay-Sachs disease.
13. beta-thalassaemia.
14. spina bifida occulta.
15. oesophageal atresia.

103

Antenatal fetal blood sampling

F 16. from the umbilical artery rather than from the umbilical vein is associated with more fetal complications.

F 17. from the placental cord insertion ensures a fetal rather than a maternal sample.

F 18. is regularly performed between 14 and 16 weeks of gestation.

T 19. has a fetal loss rate independent of the indication.

Duchenne muscular dystrophy

F 20. may be identified by measuring the maternal creatine kinase activity at 18 weeks of gestation.

F 21. only occurs when the mother carries the defective gene.

F 22. may now be effectively treated with the protein 'dystrophin'.

The following conditions would be expected to conform to the pattern of inheritance shown in Figure 5:

T 23. Duchenne muscular dystrophy.

F 24. polyposis coli.

F 25. congenital dislocation of the hip.

T 26. red–green colour blindness.

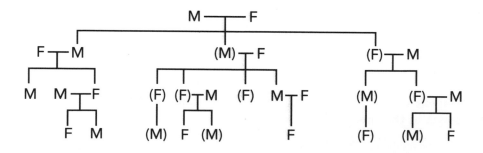

[M = normal male, (M) = affected male, F = normal female, (F) = carrier female]

Figure 5

Down syndrome due to translocation is characterised by

F 27. on average, a higher IQ than that which occurs in trisomy 21.
T 28. involvement of a chromosome of the D group.
F 29. coarctation of the aorta.
T 29. a greater paternal genetic component than trisomy 21.

The following diseases are inherited by autosomal recessive transmission:

F 30. Huntington's chorea.
T 31. infantile polycystic kidneys.
F 32. tuberous sclerosis.

The following are typically inherited as an X-linked trait:

T 31. glucose-6-phosphate dehydrogenase deficiency.
F 32. von-Willebrand's disease.
F 33. Pierre-Robin disease.

The following statements relating to toxoplasmosis and pregnancy are correct:

T 34. Severe disease in the fetus is most likely to occur if the mother acquires the infection during the first two trimesters of pregnancy.
F 35. Evidence of prior infection occurs in more than 50% of women in Britain.

Congenital rubella syndrome in the neonate

F 36. is likely to follow accidental vaccination of the mother with rubella vaccine in the first trimester.
T 37. may result in excretion of the rubella virus for more than six months.
F 38. includes intracranial calcification.

Eye damage is a recognised consequence of fetal infection with

T 39. cytomegalovirus.
T 40. *Treponema pallidum*.
T 41. the Epstein-Barr virus.

The following are recognised clinical manifestations of infection with *Listeria monocytogenes*:

T 42. neonatal pneumonia and septicaemia within five days of birth.
T 43. preterm labour associated with meconium-stained liquor.
T 44. stillbirth.

Regarding group B Streptococcus, the following statements are correct:

F 45. Antenatal antibiotic treatment of carriers reduces neonatal morbidity.
F 46. Five percent of pregnant women carry the organism.

Symptomatic intrahepatic cholestasis of pregnancy characteristically

F 47. is associated with neonatal jaundice.
T 48. is associated with premature delivery.
F 49. is unlikely to recur in a subsequent pregnancy.

The following statements regarding inflammatory bowel disease during pregnancy are correct:

T 50. Ulcerative colitis developing for the first time in pregnancy is likely to be severe.
F 51. Azathioprine therapy is associated with significant embryopathy.

Acute pulmonary thromboembolism occurring during pregnancy

F 52. is more likely to occur in women of blood group 0 than those of blood group A.
T 53. is a recognised complication of severe iron deficiency anaemia.

Phaeochromocytoma complicating pregnancy is characteristically associated with

T 54. a high output of 5-hydroxyindoleacetic acid in the urine.
T 55. impaired carbohydrate tolerance.

Asymptomatic bacteriuria in pregnancy

F 56. if untreated, is followed later in pregnancy by acute pyelonephritis in 60–70% of women.
F 57. causes preterm labour in approximately 40% of affected patients.
T 58. affects approximately 5% of pregnant women.

Features of sickle cell haemoglobin C (Hb SC) disease in pregnancy include

T 59.   fat embolus.

Concerning anaemia in pregnancy (excluding the haemoglobinopathies),

T 60.   red-cell folate estimation provides more useful information than does the plasma folate concentration.

F 61.   a microcytic blood film excludes folate deficiency.

Myotonic dystrophy

F 62.   is more commonly inherited from the father than from the mother.

T 63.   may present as polyhydramnios in pregnancy.

T 64.   is inherited as an autosomal dominant condition.

The following statements concerning cardiovascular disease and pregnancy are correct:

F 65.   Maternal deaths with Eisenmenger syndrome usually occur before delivery.

T 66.   Congenital heart disease is numerically more important than acquired heart disease as a cause of maternal mortality in Britain.

F 67.   Pregnant women are less susceptible than nonpregnant to cystic medial necrosis of the aorta.

F 68.   The maternal mortality from Eisenmenger syndrome is approximately 30%.

T 69.   When myocardial infarction occurs during pregnancy, maternal mortality exceeds 25%.

The following statements regarding pregnancy complicated by insulin-dependent diabetes mellitus are correct:

F 70.   Delivery at 38 weeks prevents respiratory distress syndrome in the baby.

T 71.   Polycythaemia is a recognised complication in the newborn.

In pregnancy complicated by insulin-dependent diabetes mellitus

F 72.   impending intrauterine death is associated with a sharp fall in maternal insulin requirements.

T 73.   persistent maternal ketosis in the absence of glycosuria indicates the need for an increase in dietary carbohydrate.

The following are recognised to cross the placenta in clinically significant quantities:

T 74. quinine.
F 75. cholestyramine.
T 76. retinoic acid derivatives.
T 77. podophyllotoxin.

The use of betamimetic drugs to inhibit the onset of premature labour is contraindicated

F 78. when treatment with tricyclic antidepressants is being given.

Prostaglandin E$_2$ for the induction of labour is contraindicated in patients with

F 79. migraine.
F 80. mitral valve disease.

The following are recognised complications of the use of an intravenous oxytocin infusion:

T 81. neonatal jaundice.
T 82. amniotic fluid embolism.
F 83. fetal hypoglycaemia.

An increased intake of folic acid is required when pregnancy is associated with

T 84. the administration of carbamazepine.
F 85. the administration of carbimazole.
T 86. maternal coeliac disease.
T 87. beta-thalassaemia.

In pregnant women aged 35 years or over there is an increased incidence of

F 88. anencephaly.
F 89. breech presentation.
T 90. dizygotic twins.

Monozygotic twinning is

F 91. familial.
F 92. associated with a common amniotic sac in about 25% of cases.
F 93. related to advanced maternal age.

Disseminated intravascular coagulation has a recognised association with

94.   placenta praevia.
95.   prolonged bed rest.

The following condition can cause reduction in uteroplacental blood flow:

96.   intermittent positive pressure hyperventilation.

Women with proteinuric pregnancy induced hypertension (pre-eclampsia) will characteristically show raised

97.   creatinine clearance.
98.   peripheral vascular resistance.

The following conditions have a recognised association with spontaneous preterm labour:

99.   teenage pregnancy.
100. maternal body mass index (BMI) below 19.

Factors characteristically associated with the spontaneous onset of premature labour include

101. oligohydramnios.
102. bicornuate uterus.

A primigravid patient is delivered by lower-segment caesarean section for fetal distress. In a second pregnancy

103. there is an increased incidence of placenta praevia.
104. the lower uterine scar should be palpated following a vaginal delivery.

Recognised complications of external cephalic version include

105. amniotic fluid embolism.
106. transient maternal hypertension.

With regard to oblique lie of the fetus,

107. at term, dorso-anterior positions are more frequent than dorso-posterior.

F 108. there is a recognised association with fetal renal agenesis.

The following statements concerning epidural blockade are correct:

T 109. Leakage of cerebrospinal fluid is a recognised cause of headache.
T 110. Hypotension is a greater hazard in a patient on antihypertensive therapy.

The secretion of breast milk is decreased by the administration of

F 111. oxytocin.
F 112. metoclopramide.
F 113. norethisterone acetate.
F 114. methadone.

Perinatal mortality in the United Kingdom

T 115. is associated with low-birthweight (less than 2.5 kg) babies in over 60% of cases.
F 116. is lower in babies of mothers who are primiparous.

The Report on Confidential Enquiries into Maternal Deaths in the United Kingdom (1994–1996) showed that:

F 117. there are more maternal deaths from road traffic accidents than from obstetric haemorrhage.
T 118. the most common cause of death in hypertensive disorders of pregnancy is cerebral haemorrhage.
T 119. in women aged over 40 years the risk of maternal death is four times greater than in women under 25 years.
T 120. death from amniotic fluid embolism is more common after assisted delivery.

With regard to non-immune hydrops fetalis,

F 121. it is responsible for 3% of all perinatal morbidity.
F 122. there is a 20% risk of chromosomal abnormality.

Congenital dislocation of the hip is characteristically

T 123. more common in girls than boys.
F 124. bilateral in more than 50% of cases.
T 125. associated with persistent breech presentation.

The incidence of the following are increased in preterm neonates:

F 126. meconium ileus.
T 127. polyuria.

Neonatal jaundice appearing 12 hours after delivery is a recognised feature of

F 128. sickle cell disease.
F 129. physiological haemolysis.
F 130. atresia of the bile ducts.

In the management of infants with suspected rhesus haemolytic disease,

F 131. ABO compatible rhesus positive blood should be used for transfusion.

Recognised causes of purulent vaginal discharge in a two-year-old girl include

F 132. urinary tract infection.
F 133. threadworm infection.

In non-mosaic Turner's syndrome

T 134. the external genitalia are normal.
T 135. there is a low occipital hairline.

In the complete androgen insensitivity syndrome (testicular feminisation)

T 136. a familial incidence is recognised.
F 137. following gonadectomy, hormone replacement therapy is not indicated.

Recognised effects of the administration of danazol include

T 138. synergism with the anticoagulant effect of the biscoumarins (warfarin sodium).
F 139. the development of fibrocystic mastitis.
T 140. suppression of sex hormone-binding globulin (SHBG).

The following is correctly paired with a recognised clinical association:

F 141. Inappropriate secretion of antidiuretic hormone : hypernatraemia.

There is a recognised association between hirsutism and

F 142. dysgerminoma of the ovary.

In a 25-year-old woman, serum follicle-stimulating hormone concentration is characteristically raised in

F 143. acromegaly.
F 144. the presence of a Krukenberg tumour.

The serum luteinising hormone concentration is raised in

F 145. anorexia nervosa.
T 146. ovarian agenesis.

The menstrual irregularities that characteristically occur in highly athletic women

T 147. can return to normal as a result of rest without an increase in the body mass index.
F 148. are not related to stress induced by competition.
T 149. lead to osteoporosis when the amenorrhoea is prolonged (over 12 months).

Congenital adrenal hyperplasia due to 21-hydroxylase deficiency is characteristically associated with excessive production of

T 150. 17-alpha-hydroxyprogesterone.
T 151. androstenedione.
T 152. adrenocorticotrophic hormone.

Recognised causes of hyperprolactinaemia include

T 153. administration of thyrotrophin-releasing hormone (TRH).
T 154. lesions of the pituitary stalk.
F 155. thyrotoxicosis.
T 156. acromegaly.

A 30-year-old woman, who had been taking the combined oral contraceptive pill for four years, stopped it one year ago as she wished to become pregnant. Since then, her periods have occurred every 9–12 weeks. On examination, she is thin and anxious. She measures 1.52 m in height and weighs 41.5 kg, giving her a body mass index of 18 (normal range 19–26). On examination, the abdomen and pelvis are normal. Her partner has a normal semen analysis. In relation to this patient the following statements are correct:

157. The delay in conception is likely to be significantly related to her long-term use of the contraceptive pill.
158. Ovarian biopsy should be carried out at the time of laparoscopy.

Recognised associations exist between primary dysmenorrhoea and

159. endometriosis.
160. anovulatory cycles.

The following statements concerning the intrauterine contraceptive device (IUCD) are correct:

161. Insertion immediately after first-trimester termination of pregnancy is associated with an increase in the expulsion rate.
162. Inert devices should be removed after a maximum of ten years.
163. Pregnancy is most likely to occur in the early months after insertion.
164. Actinomycosis-like organisms are more commonly found with inert devices.

Following vasectomy,

165. the failure rate is approximately 2/1000.
166. sperm autoantibodies develop in at least 40% of patients.
167. epididymo-orchitis is the most common immediate side effect.

Recognised effects of progestogen only oral contraceptive therapy include

168. inhibition of ovulation in over 90% of subjects.
169. poor cycle control.

The following are recommended techniques for termination of pregnancy:

170. At ten weeks of gestation: oral mifepristone followed by a prostaglandin analogue.

T 171. At 12 weeks of gestation: gemeprost pessary followed by suction curettage.

Characteristic features of ectopic gestation include

F 172. occurrence in the outer third of the fallopian tube.
F 173. coexisting infection with *Chlamydia trachomatis*.

Hydatidiform mole (chorioadenoma destruens)

F 174. characteristically produces luteinising hormone.
T 175. is typically associated with theca lutein ovarian cysts.

With respect to the management of choriocarcinoma,

T 176. successful chemotherapy is followed by the return of fertility in most young women.

In the male partner of an infertile couple

F 177. azoospermia with a normal plasma follicle-stimulating hormone concentration indicates failure of the germinal epithelium.
T 178. cigarette smoking (more than ten in a day) impairs sperm motility.

Azoospermia associated with high concentrations of serum follicle-stimulating hormone are characteristically found in the presence of

T 179. a 47XXY karyotype.
F 180. congenital absence of the vas deferens.
F 181. bilateral varicocele.

Concerning intracytoplasmic sperm injection (ICSI),

F 182. it results in a higher proportion of male offspring compared with natural conception.
F 183. in oligospermic males there is no increased incidence of Y chromosome deletions.
F 184. sperm retrieved from the epididymis result in higher fertilisation rates than those from an ejaculate.
T 185. use of immotile sperm results in lower fertilisation rates.

Complications of clomifene citrate therapy include

T 186. visual disturbance.
T 187. ascites.

T 188. hot flushes.
T 189. hair loss.

In a patient with chlamydial infection

T 190. lymphogranuloma venereum is a recognised clinical presentation.
F 191. neonatal conjunctivitis appears in the first 48 hours after birth.

Untreated female genital tuberculosis is characteristically associated with

F 192. recurrent miscarriage.
F 193. psoas abscess.
T 194. lack of symptoms for long periods of time.

Pelvic abscess is a recognized complication of

T 195. pyometra.
T 196. radiotherapy for carcinoma of the cervix.
T 197. ulcerative colitis.

When treating women with heavy menstrual bleeding,

T 198. the use of the combined oral contraceptive pill is associated with a lower mortality than is hysterectomy regardless of age or smoking habits.
F 199. the combined oral contraceptive pill restores bleeding to normal in 25% of patients with fibroids.

Recognised features of the postmenopause include

T 200. atrophic trigonitis of the bladder.
F 201. fall in plasma calcium concentration.

Recognised causes of postmenopausal bleeding in women not receiving hormone replacement therapy include

T 202. thecoma of the ovary.
F 203. cirrhosis of the liver.

Enterocele

F 204. is characteristically associated with difficulty in emptying the rectum.
T 205. can be congenital.
T 206. is more common than uterine prolapse in nulliparous women.

Genuine stress incontinence

F 207. occurs in about 5% of nulliparous women.
F 208. is more common in the second half of the menstrual cycle.

The following drugs are recognised as useful in the management of detrusor instability:

F 209. bethanechol.
F 210. phenoxybenzamine.
T 211. imipramine.

During conventional urodynamic studies (dual-channel subtracted cystometry with simultaneous pressure–flow measurements) in a normal woman

F 212. involuntary detrusor contractions are seen after the first sensation of filling is appreciated.
F 213. voiding pressure should be greater than 80 cm water.
T 214. the detrusor pressure rise during filling should be less than 15 cm water.

Pruritus vulvae is a recognised symptom of

T 215. Taenia saginata infestation.
F 216. achlorhydria.
T 217. Behcet's syndrome.
T 218. psoriasis.

With regard to the vulva,

T 219. pruritus is a feature of vulval intraepithelial neoplasia (VIN3).
F 220. malignant change occurs in more than 45% of cases of hyperplastic atypia.

The following are appropriate for the treatment of vaginal intraepithelial neoplasia (VAIN):

T 221. local surgical excision.
T 222. superficial radiotherapy.
F 223. application of topical 5-fluorouracil.

The following statements concerning the fallopian tube are correct:

F 224. X-ray hysterosalpingography is the most accurate way of testing tubal patency.

F 225. Pyosalpinx is a common sequel to post-abortion infection.
T 226. It is the commonest site for genital tuberculosis.

A 38-year-old woman who has completed her family has a second-degree uterine prolapse. Her cervical smear is abnormal and colposcopy and biopsy shows cervical intraepithelial neoplasia stage 3 (CIN3). Appropriate management includes

F 227. urgent cone biopsy.
F 228. local ablative treatment of the cervix.

A 25-year-old woman with two children has had three borderline smears in the last 18 months. Colposcopic examination reveals no abnormality and endocervical brush smears are reported as normal. The following procedures are appropriate:

F 229. loop diathermy excision.
T 230. punch biopsy.
F 231. cryotherapy.

At colposcopic assessment of the cervix

F 232. the cervix should be painted with a 10% acetic acid solution.
F 233. the presence of mosaicism is an indication for cone biopsy.

Factors that are considered to predispose to the development of carcinoma of the endometrium include

F 234. previous radiation-induced menopause.
F 235. adrenal hyperplasia.
F 236. hilus cell tumour.
T 237. tamoxifen therapy.

The incidence of extrapelvic recurrence of endometrial carcinoma following hysterectomy is significantly reduced by

F 238. the long-term administration of oral oestrogen.
F 239. external irradiation of the pelvic side walls.
F 240. vaginal vault irradiation with caesium.

High levels of serum CA125 are a common feature of

T 241. advanced endometrial adenocarcinoma.
T 242. ovarian endometrioma.

Pseudomyxoma peritonei

F 243. requires leakage from a parent cyst for the development of the condition.
F 244. is characteristically associated with intestinal obstruction.
F 245. is associated with pleural effusion.

In the treatment of ovarian cancer

F 246. second-line chemotherapy often produces dramatic remission of the disease.
F 247. chemotherapy is not indicated in stage I disease.

Granulosa-cell ovarian tumours

F 248. when malignant characteristically lead to recurrence within two years of the original diagnosis.
F 249. are bilateral in more than 20% of cases.
T 250. can occur at any age.

The following statements concerning female cancers in the UK are correct:

T 251. The proportion of women with cancer of the endometrium who will die from the disease is approximately 40%.
T 252. The lifetime risk of a woman developing breast cancer is approximately 10%.

Recognised causes of cystic swellings within the female breast include

T 253. duct carcinoma.
F 254. Paget's disease.

The following statement relating to diagnostic hysteroscopy is correct:

F 255. Uterine distension is safely produced with a laparoscopy CO_2 insufflator.

The following statements regarding transcervical resection of the endometrium are correct:

T 256. Carbon dioxide should not be used to distend the uterus.
F 257. It is effective contraception.
F 258. Fluid overload is the most common complication.

Five days after total abdominal hysterectomy, a patient develops a profuse watery vaginal discharge. The following investigation would assist in reaching a diagnosis:

F 259. estimation of the potassium level in the fluid.

T 260. intravenous urography.

The following statements concerning intestinal obstruction are correct:

T 261. Gas demonstrated throughout the small and large bowel makes diagnosis of postoperative ileus more likely than mechanical obstruction.

T 262. Intra-abdominal adhesions are the most common cause of obstruction of the small intestine in adults.

F 263. Absence of bowel sounds excludes mechanical obstruction.

Postoperative pelvic deep vein thrombosis occurs more commonly

T 264. on the left than the right.

F 265. in patients of blood group O.

T 266. when there are superficial leg varicosities.

September 2000

A recognised association exists between polyhydramnios and

T 1. anencephaly.
T 2. an imperforate anus in the fetus.
F 3. fetal polycystic kidneys.

The following have a recognised association with transverse lie of the fetus in late pregnancy or labour:

F 4. microcephaly.
T 5. high parity.
T 6. a bicornuate uterus.

The following statements concerning preterm labour are correct:

T 7. Urinary tract infection is associated with a greater risk.
F 8. Babies weighing between 500 g and 1000 g should be delivered by caesarean section.
F 9. Women with a history of subfertility have an increased risk.

The following statements concerning the bony pelvis are correct:

T 10. The angle of inclination of the pelvic brim is greater in Afro-Caribbean than in Caucasian women.
T 11. In the anthropoid type of female pelvis, the anteroposterior diameter of the inlet is significantly greater than the transverse diameter.
T 12. A straight sacrum is associated with a narrow subpubic angle.
F 13. The sacrosciatic notch is significantly wider in an android pelvis.
T 14. The female pelvis is characteristically shallower than the male pelvis.

The following are recognised to cross the placenta in clinically significant quantities:

T 15. indomethacin.
T 16. lithium.

120

F 17. cholestyramine.
T 18. podophyllotoxin.

Amniocentesis

T 19. carries an increased risk of orthopaedic deformity as a sequel.
F 20. has a risk of chorioamnionitis in 3–5% of cases.

The following are recognised complications of the use of an intravenous oxytocin infusion:

T 21. neonatal jaundice.
F 22. maternal hyperglycaemia.

Compared with vacuum extraction, a Kielland forceps delivery is associated with an increased incidence of

F 23. neonatal jaundice.
F 24. subgaleal (sub-aponeurotic) haematoma.
T 25. facial palsy.

Congenital infection with cytomegalovirus

T 26. is associated with intracerebral calcification.
T 27. is associated with fetal growth restriction.
T 28. is a recognised cause of microcephaly.
T 29. can be detected by culture of the infant's urine.

Phaeochromocytoma complicating pregnancy is characteristically associated with

F 30. secretion of dopamine.
T 31. a high output of 5-hydroxyindoleacetic acid in the urine.
T 32. impaired carbohydrate tolerance.
T 33. precordial pain.

Disseminated intravascular coagulation has a recognised association with

T 34. placenta praevia.
F 35. multiple pregnancy.
F 36. iron deficiency anaemia.
F 37. prolonged bed rest.

Acute pulmonary thromboembolism occurring during pregnancy

T 38.   has a recognised association with advancing maternal age.
T 39.   is a recognised complication of severe iron deficiency anaemia.

Concerning ultrasound in pregnancy,

F 40.   ultrasound markers may be detected during a second-trimester scan in 70% of fetuses with Down syndrome.
T 41.   the risk of aneuploidy increases when there are two or more markers present.
T 42.   most fetuses with a nuchal translucency of 2.5 mm or more are normal.

Women with proteinuric pregnancy-induced hypertension (pre-eclampsia) will characteristically show raised

F 43.   creatinine clearance.
F 44.   platelet concentration.

Asymptomatic bacteriuria in pregnancy

F 45.   if untreated, is followed later in pregnancy by acute pyelonephritis in 60–70% of women.
F 46.   is associated with raised levels of maternal serum alphafetoprotein at 16 weeks of gestation.

Patients with acute pyelonephritis in pregnancy

T 47.   are at risk of developing endotoxic shock.

In amniotic fluid embolism,

F 48.   detection of trophoblastic cells in the peripheral circulation is pathognomonic.
F 49.   up to 15% of patients present with the complications of a bleeding diathesis as the first indication of the condition.
F 50.   maternal death occurs in over 80% of reported cases.
F 51.   symptoms characteristically occur before the onset of labour.

The congenital rubella syndrome

F 52.   can be prevented by the administration of immunoglobulin to an infected mother during pregnancy.
T 53.   is associated with neonatal persistent ductus arteriosus.
T 54.   includes neonatal purpura.

The following is a recognised effect of the administration of beta-sympathomimetics to the mother:

F 55. decreased maternal blood insulin concentration.

When pregnancy occurs in a woman over the age of 35 years, there is a recognised increase in the

F 56. incidence of pregnancy prolonged beyond 40 weeks.
T 57. frequency of multiple pregnancy.
F 58. frequency of fetal neural tube defects.

In a child with Down syndrome there is a recognised association with

T 59. an atrial septal defect.
T 60. congenital duodenal atresia.
T 61. hypotonia.

The following diseases are inherited by autosomal recessive transmission:

F 62. Huntington's chorea.
F 63. myotonic dystrophy.
T 64. infantile polycystic kidneys.
T 65. galactosaemia.
F 66. achondroplasia.

The incidence of the following is increased in the preterm neonate:

F 67. meconium ileus.

Haemolytic disease of the newborn is

T 68. characterised by erythroblasts in the cord blood.
T 69. associated with a positive direct Coombs test in the cord blood.
T 70. characterised by jaundice present at birth.

Concerning shoulder dystocia,

T 71. brachial plexus injury involves cervical nerve roots 5 and 6 more frequently than 7 and 8.
T 72. for a given birth weight it occurs more often in babies of diabetic mothers.

The following conditions would be expected to conform to the pattern of inheritance shown in Figure 6:

73. adrenal hyperplasia.
74. haemophilia A (classical).
75. congenital dislocation of the hip.

Congenital malformations in the fetus are more common after the following maternal infections during pregnancy:

76. mumps.
77. genital herpes simplex virus type II.
78. malaria.
79. toxoplasmosis.

The following disorders are correctly associated with the mode of inheritance:

80. von Recklinghausen's disease (neurofibromatosis) : autosomal dominant.
81. Tay-Sachs disease : autosomal recessive.

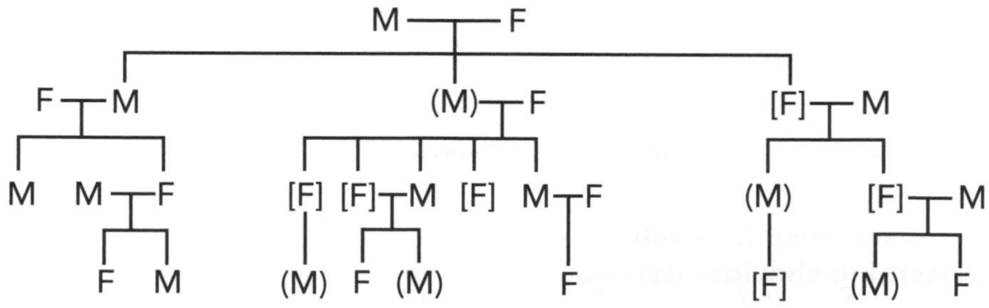

M = normal male, (M) = affected male, F = normal female, [F] = carrier female

Figure 6

124

Sacral agenesis

T 82. is a recognised complication of propylthiouracil treatment in the first trimester.
F 83. is a recognised complication of fetal toxoplasmosis.
F 84. has an association with an elevated maternal serum alphafetoprotein concentration.
T 85. is related to poor glucose homeostasis in the first trimester.

The following statements concerning fetal hydrocephalus are correct:

T 86. Chromosomal abnormalities are found in less than 15% of cases.
T 87. It has a causal association with fetal viral infections.
T 88. It may be a result of Arnold–Chiari malformation.

With regard to anencephaly,

T 89. small adrenal glands are characteristic.
F 90. renal agenesis is commonly associated.

Maternal administration of glucocorticoids, used to prevent respiratory distress syndrome in the newborn,

T 91. is contraindicated between 26 and 32 weeks of gestation in the presence of ruptured membranes.
T 92. is most effective if given within 48 hours before delivery.
F 93. has not been shown to reduce the incidence of the condition.
F 94. is unnecessary if neonatal surfactant treatment is available.

Regarding the fetal heart,

F 95. a four-chamber view at ultrasound examination detects approximately 60% of serious structural abnormalities.
T 96. more than 10% of fetuses with persistent antepartum bradycardia have a structural cardiac abnormality.

Duchenne muscular dystrophy

F 97. may be identified by measuring the maternal creatine kinase activity at 18 weeks of gestation.
T 98. is the commonest X-linked cause of reduced life expectancy in males.
F 99. only occurs when the mother carries the defective gene.
F 100. is less common following donor insemination.

For a pregnant woman, the risk of having a fetus affected by Down syndrome

T 101. who is born at term is, at a maternal age of thirty-five years, approximately 1/360 births.

T 102. increases if serum beta-human chorionic gonadotrophin concentration is elevated at 16 weeks of pregnancy.

T 103. increases if the woman has had a previous child with Down syndrome.

F 104. is increased if a single stomach bubble is identified on ultrasound.

T 105. at ten weeks, is approximately double that of having an affected live baby.

Following vaginal delivery of the first twin, in the delivery of the second twin

F 106. when the head is not engaged, the ventouse should not be used.

T 107. external cephalic version should be considered.

F 108. internal podalic version is no longer an acceptable procedure.

Drugs considered suitable to be prescribed to the breastfeeding mother include

T 109. phenytoin.

T 110. propylthiouracil.

Breastfeeding is compromised by

T 111. dopamine agonists.

F 112. metoclopramide.

F 113. depo-medroxyprogesterone acetate.

The following conditions and features occurring in pregnancy are appropriately paired:

T 114. mitral stenosis : orthopnoea.

F 115. hyperthyroidism : acne.

T 116. Hodgkin's disease : fever.

In a prospective, blind study of a possible new method of antenatal screening for a particular fetal disorder, 60,000 consecutive pregnant women were recruited and tested. One hundred of the fetuses were found to be affected. The test had a sensitivity of 90% and a specificity of 95%. Based on this study, the following statements are correct:

F 117. A woman with a positive test has a 10% chance of having an affected child.

F 118. The results demonstrate that the test fulfils the criteria set by the World Health Organization for screening.

F 119. 95% of affected cases had a positive screening test.

F 120. The false positive rate can be calculated using Fisher's exact test.

With regard to premature ovarian failure,

F 121. it should be differentiated from resistant ovary syndrome by ovarian biopsy.

F 122. serum concentrations of follicle-stimulating hormone greater than 40 iu/l indicate permanent ovarian failure.

F 123. it is associated with an increased risk of ovarian malignancy.

T 124. it occurs in approximately 1% of women under 40 years of age.

T 125. the major genetic cause is ovarian dysgenesis.

Changes in the serum compatible with a premature menopause include

F 126. an increase in prolactin concentration.

T 127. an increase in calcium concentration. ?

T 128. an increase in cholesterol concentration.

Characteristic features of the androgen insensitivity (testicular feminisation) syndrome in an adult include

T 129. a family history of the condition.

T 130. inguinal hernia.

F 131. the 47XXY karyotype.

F 132. breast hypoplasia.

F 133. hypospadias.

Secondary amenorrhoea is a recognised feature of

T 134. Addison's disease.

T 135. chronic renal failure.

T 136. beta-thalassaemia major.

T 137. Down syndrome.

Precocious puberty

F 138. of the central (constitutional) type is more common in boys than in girls.

T 139. is a recognised feature of polyostotic fibrous dysplasia (Albright's syndrome).

F 140. has a recognised association with benign teratoma of the ovary.

T 141. has a recognised association with juvenile hypothyroidism.

In patients with Turner syndrome

T 142. pregnancy may be achieved by assisted conception using donated ova.

T 143. uterine bleeding can be induced with cyclical oestrogen/progestogen therapy.

T 144. breast development will be poor.

A thirty-year-old woman of 1.6 m height complains of secondary amenorrhoea and hot flushes. Her periods began at the age of 12 years and were regular until eight months ago, when they stopped suddenly. After the birth of her second child (six years ago) she had a postpartum haemorrhage, necessitating a three-unit blood transfusion. Four years ago, she was diagnosed as having insulin-dependent diabetes, which has been difficult to control. As a result of this and her husband's unemployment she has lost 7 kg to her present weight of 45 kg (body mass index 17.59). Her blood chemistry results include: 17-beta oestradiol 80 pmol/l; follicle-stimulating 44 iu/l; cortisol 130 nmol/l. On the information given above, the following statements are correct:

F 145. Weight gain of about 5 kg will almost certainly lead to return of menstruation.

F 146. Successful stabilisation of her diabetes is likely to result in a return of menstruation.

T 147. The clinical picture is consistent with autoimmune ovarian failure.

T 148. Without treatment she is at risk of developing premature osteoporosis.

F 149. A diagnosis of panhypopituitarism has not been excluded.

Recognised causes of galactorrhoea include

T 150. primary hypothyroidism.

T 151. pituitary stalk section.

T 152. chronic renal failure.

F 153. administration of spironolactone.

F 154. administration of danazol.

In a patient with inappropriate lactation associated with secondary amenorrhoea,

F   155.   bi-temporal hemianopia would be expected in about 25% of patients.
F   156.   an increased plasma progesterone concentration would be expected.
T   157.   the administration of methyldopa is a recognised cause.
F   158.   anorexia nervosa is a recognised association.

With regard to the finding of a pelvic mass in an adolescent girl,

F   159.   there is a recognised association between renal tract anomalies and ovarian tumours.
T   160.   subsequent ultrasound assessment showing a solid ovarian tumour is suggestive of a dysgerminoma.
T   161.   the diagnosis of haematocolpos may be made clinically.
F   162.   the commonest type of ovarian cyst is an epithelial cystadenoma.

Azoospermia associated with high concentrations of follicle stimulating hormone is characteristically found in the presence of

T   163.   Klinefelter syndrome.
T   164.   testicular atrophy.
F   165.   congenital absence of the vas deferens.
F   166.   bilateral varicocele.
F   167.   a previous vasectomy.

Oligozoospermia has a recognised association with

F   168.   bronchiectasis.
T   169.   sulfasalazine therapy.

Sperm transport through the cervical canal may be impaired by

F   170.   the presence of *Escherichia coli* in the cervical mucus.
F   171.   the preovulatory surge of luteinising hormone.
T   172.   clomifene citrate.

Recognised effects of progestogen-only oral contraceptive therapy include

F   173.   inhibition of ovulation in over 90% of subjects.
T   174.   poor cycle control.
F   175.   fibroadenosis of the breast.
F   176.   intrahepatic cholestasis.

The following statements relating to sexual dysfunction are correct:

T 177. A complaint of recurrent vaginal discharge, with no detectable pathology, is a recognised presentation of psychosexual difficulties.

F 178. Patients with psychosexual problems commonly have a psychiatric illness.

Procedures of value in the diagnosis of gonorrhoea in the female include

F 179. culture of a high vaginal swab.

F 180. the naked-eye examination of the vaginal discharge.

T 181. culture of a swab from the anal canal.

The toxic shock syndrome has a recognised association with

T 182. a fever of 39°C or more.

T 183. diarrhoea.

T 184. a generalised macular erythema.

F 185. isolation of the group B streptococcus.

Enterocele

F 186. is characteristically associated with difficulty in emptying the rectum.

T 187. can be congenital.

T 188. is a recognised complication of vaginal hysterectomy. (?)

F 189. is characteristically associated with painful defaecation.

Genuine stress incontinence of urine

F 190. improves during pregnancy.

F 191. is caused by an overactive detrusor muscle.

F 192. can only be diagnosed by urodynamic investigation.

T 193. is improved by elevation of the urethrovesical angle.

Features characteristically associated with an imperforate vagina in a girl aged 16 years include

F 194. absence of secondary sexual characteristics.

F 195. a pelvic kidney.

F 196. short stature.

F 197. closed spina bifida.

T 198. the presence of pelvic endometriosis.

Pyometra is a recognised complication of

F 199. acute endometritis.
T 200. cone biopsy of the cervix.
F 201. the presence of an intrauterine contraceptive device.

The following statements concerning trophoblastic disease are correct:

T 202. Choriocarcinoma may be accompanied by clinical evidence of thyrotoxicosis.
T 203. There is a significant increase in incidence beyond the age of 40 years.
T 204. The prognosis is influenced by the patient's ABO blood group.
F 205. The tissue karyotype is characteristically 46XX.

Characteristic features of primary spasmodic dysmenorrhoea include

T 206. relief of pain by mefenamic acid.
F 207. a delayed menarche.
F 208. raised concentrations of serum prolactin.
F 209. an association with uterine hypoplasia.

Noninvasive (complete) hydatidiform mole

T 210. has a ten times increased risk of occurring in a subsequent pregnancy compared with women who have no history of molar pregnancy.
F 211. occurs most frequently in a first pregnancy.

The following predispose to the development of endometrial carcinoma:

F 212. adrenal hyperplasia.
T 213. tamoxifen therapy.
T 214. polycystic ovary syndrome.

Endometrial hyperplasia is characteristically associated with

T 215. anovulatory cycles.
F 216. hyperthyroidism.
F 217. vaginal adenosis.
F 218. hyperprolactinaemia.
F 219. the use of intrauterine contraceptive devices.

Uterine curettage

F 220. is essential in the investigation of secondary amenorrhoea.
F 221. is curative in about 50% of cases of menorrhagia of unknown aetiology.

In women with idiopathic heavy menstrual bleeding,

F 222. there is abnormal platelet function in the uterine blood vessels.

In the international (FIGO) staging of ovarian carcinoma

F 223. stage II carcinoma is limited to the ovaries.
T 224. secondary deposits in the omentum indicate stage III.
T 225. ascites can be present in stage I.

Ovarian tumours which secrete oestrogens include

F 226. endometrioma.
F 227. dysgerminoma.
T 228. granulosa-cell tumour.

Bilateral oophorectomy in premenopausal women

F 229. is indicated at the time of radical hysterectomy for cervical cancer in young women.
T 230. is associated with an increase of vertebral collapse in later life.
T 231. is associated with an increased incidence of coronary heart disease.
F 232. is required in women under the age of 30 years, with stage Ia ovarian cancer.
F 233. is indicated in patients with 45X gonadal dysgenesis.

Krukenberg tumours

F 234. contain Kupffer cells.
T 235. are characteristically bilateral.

Ovarian neoplasms occurring under the age of 20 years

F 236. require the removal of the contralateral ovary if a malignant germ-cell tumour is diagnosed.
F 267. are most commonly epithelial in type.

Ovarian thecomas

T 238. are typically benign.
F 239. are characteristically bilateral.
F 240. characteristically occur before puberty.
T 241. are a recognised cause of Meig syndrome.
T 242. have a recognised association with endometrial hyperplasia.

Cisplatinum

F 243. usually causes alopecia.
T 244. is ototoxic.
T 245. seldom produces severe myelosuppression.

Noncystic lesions of the vulva include

F 246. hidradenoma.
T 247. accessory breast tissue.
F 248. Nabothian follicles.

Recognised causes of vulval ulceration include

T 249. lymphogranuloma venereum (*Chlamydia trachomatis*).
F 250. lichen sclerosus.
T 251. Behcet's syndrome.
T 252. tuberculosis.
T 253. actinomycosis.

Routine examination of a cervical smear can identify the presence of

T 254. *Trichomonas vaginalis*.
F 255. *Chlamydia trachomatis*.
F 256. *Neisseria gonorrhoea*.
T 257. *Candida albicans*.

The following are correctly paired with a recognised clinical association:

F 258. inappropriate secretion of antidiuretic hormone : hypernatraemia.
F 259. carcinoma of ovary : hypocalcaemia.
T 260. choriocarcinoma : hyperthyroidism.
T 261. uterine fibromyomata : polycythaemia.
T 262. adrenal carcinoma : hirsutism.

The following disorders are correctly linked with a recognised association:

F 263. polycystic ovary syndrome : raised serum sex hormone-binding globulin concentration.
T 264. isolated gonadotrophin deficiency : anosmia.
T 265. pure gonadal dysgenesis : 46XY karyotype.
F 266. complete androgen insensitivity syndrome : hirsutism.
T 267. Klinefelter syndrome : impotence.

The following conditions are correctly paired with a characteristic laboratory finding:

T 268. congenital adrenal hyperplasia (21-hydroxylase deficiency) : elevated serum 17-alphahydroxy-progesterone concentration.
F 269. anorexia nervosa : elevated serum follicle-stimulating hormone concentration.

March 2001

The following statements relating to pregnancy in a 38-year-old woman are correct:

F 1. Her risk of having a child with a neural tube defect is ten times greater than at the age of 18 years.

F 2. Chorionic villus sampling will allow the diagnosis of a neural tube defect.

T 3. Her risk of having a child with Down syndrome is less than 1%.

Down syndrome

T 4. has an incidence in the United Kingdom of approximately one in 700 live births.

F 5. is more commonly due to translocation than to non-dysjunction.

The following disorders are correctly associated with the mode of inheritance:

T 6. glucose-6-phosphate dehydrogenase deficiency : X-linked recessive.

F 7. polycystic disease of the kidneys (adult form) : multifactorial.

T 8. von Willebrand's disease : autosomal dominant.

Methods of value to distinguish the fetus with intrauterine growth restriction from that of uncertain gestational age include

T 9. increasing ratio of head to abdominal circumference measured by ultrasound.

F 10. measurement of fetal breathing activity.

F 11. a single ultrasonic measurement of the biparietal diameter at 37 weeks.

Recognised causes of non-immune hydrops fetalis include

T 12. alpha-thalassaemia.

F 13. renal agenesis.

An increased risk of fetal malformation is associated with

F 14. the presence of a single umbilical vein.
F 15. smoking 20 cigarettes or more a day.
F 16. rubella vaccination in the first trimester of pregnancy.

The fetal alcohol syndrome

F 17. is associated with an increased incidence of postmaturity.
T 18. seldom occurs with alcohol ingestion by the mother of under eight units per week (one unit = one glass of wine).
F 19. is reversed by a high intake of vitamins.

A geneticist notices with concern that a striking similarity in appearance exists between his son and a male neighbour. The geneticist would be reassured that he, and not the neighbour, is the true father of the child if

F 20. the neighbour's blood group is A rhesus positive and the son's is B rhesus negative.
? F 21. both the neighbour and the son have haemophilia A.
? T 22. the neighbour has cystic fibrosis.

The administration of corticosteroids is appropriate management in pregnancies affected by

T 23. hyperemesis gravidarum.
T 24. triplets.
T 25. systemic lupus erythematosus.

A woman presents at 38 weeks of gestation with right iliac fossa pain. Likely causes include

F 26. acute salpingitis.
F 27. constipation.

Likely complications of fibroids during pregnancy include

F 28. precipitate labour.
F 29. fetal growth restriction.

Factors predisposing to placental abruption include

F 30. pregnancy associated with an intrauterine contraceptive device.
T 31. homocysteinuria.

Complications of placental abruption include

T 32.   postpartum haemorrhage.
F 33.   folic acid deficiency.

The following statements regarding a parous rhesus negative, unsensitised woman who is pregnant by a new partner who is rhesus positive (D-heterozygous) are correct:

T 34.   Group O rhesus negative blood crossmatched against the mother's serum should be used if intrafetal transfusion is indicated.
T 35.   There is a 50% chance that her baby will be rhesus negative.

In a woman with a primary cytomegalovirus (CMV) infection in pregnancy

F 36.   there is a more than 50% chance of her delivering a baby with CMV-related damage.
F 37.   there is less than a 1% chance of the baby having serious long term sequelae.
F 38.   antenatal treatment reduces the risk of neonatal complications.

The following statements regarding toxoplasmosis and pregnancy are correct:

T 39.   The incidence of infection in the UK is approximately 2/1000 pregnancies.
T 40.   Spiramycin is used in the treatment of in utero toxoplasma infections.
F 41.   Toxoplasma gondii is a cause of recurrent miscarriage.

The following maternal infections may be transmitted to the newborn as a result of vaginal delivery:

T 42.   Human papillomavirus.
T 43.   Trichomonas vaginalis.
T 44.   Candida albicans.

In patients with human immunodeficiency virus (HIV) infection

F 45.   the rate of transmission to the fetus in a seropositive mother is over 50%.
T 46.   in the UK, intravenous drug abusers account for less than 10–15% of cases.
F 47.   pregnancy may accelerate the development of AIDS in seropositive women.

A 24-year-old woman is seen at the antenatal clinic in the tenth week of her second pregnancy. She reports that one week previously her two-year-old daughter had a generalised skin rash, which had been diagnosed as rubella. The patient has no memory of herself having had German measles. Serological testing shows the presence of rubella antibodies at a low titre of 1:8. From this information,

48. pooled immunoglobulin should be given, if maternal infection is suspected.
49. congenital anomalies in an affected fetus include cataract.
50. the serological test result confirms recent maternal infection.
51. the test should be repeated the following week.

Pregnancy exacerbates the clinical features associated with

52. sarcoidosis.
53. sickle cell haemoglobinopathy.
54. cutaneous neurofibromatosis.
55. peptic ulceration.
56. Eisenmenger syndrome.

The following statements concerning drug therapy in severe pregnancy-induced hypertension are correct:

57. Methyldopa does not cross the placenta.
58. Treatment with methyldopa should be limited to dosages less than 2 g per day.
59. Headache is a recognised side effect of hydralazine.
60. Labetalol is a combined alpha- and beta-adrenergic blocking agent.

The following statements about drug treatment in eclampsia are correct:

61. Maternal administration of intravenous diazepam characteristically causes diminution of fetal heart rate variation.
62. Neonatal respiratory depression is a recognised complication of magnesium sulphate overdosage.
63. Magnesium sulphate may be administered by the intramuscular route.

Regarding peripartum cardiomyopathy,

64. cerebral embolisation is a major cause of morbidity.
65. cardiac transplantation is inappropriate.

F   66.   the mortality rate within the first year is greater than 80%.
T   67.   anticoagulation is required.

The following statements regarding epilepsy complicating pregnancy are correct:

T   68.   Pregnant women with a history of epilepsy who do not require anticonvulsant therapy have an increased risk of fetal malformation.
F   69.   Breastfeeding is contraindicated in women taking anticonvulsants.

The following complications of pregnancy or the puerperium are correctly paired:

T   70.   Idiopathic thrombocytopenic purpura : primary postpartum haemorrhage.
T   71.   Sickle cell disease : pregnancy-induced hypertension.   [?]

In pregnancy complicated by maternal insulin-dependent diabetes mellitus

T   72.   the risk of intrauterine death of the fetus is greatest during the last four weeks of pregnancy.
T   73.   the insulin requirement may decrease during the first trimester.
T   74.   a normal HbAlc level is associated with a low risk of fetal abnormality.

In sickle cell disease associated with pregnancy

T   75.   the perinatal mortality in the UK is approximately four times greater than that of matched pregnancies without sickle cell disease.
F   76.   vitamin C supplements should be given.
T   77.   iron deficiency is rare.

In relation to monozygotic twin pregnancy

T   78.   'situs inversus' occurs more commonly than in the general population.
T   79.   acute polyhydramnios is more common than in dizygotic twin pregnancy.

External cephalic version after 37 completed weeks of gestation

T   80.   is a recognised cause of fetal bradycardia.
T   81.   is likely to lead to transient maternal hypertension.
F   82.   should only be performed using tocolytic agents.

The following drugs, administered in therapeutic dosage during the third trimester of pregnancy, are correctly paired with a recognised adverse effect in the fetus or neonate:

83. phenytoin : coagulation defects.
84. primaquine : methaemoglobinaemia.
85. heparin : coagulation defects.

The following are characteristically associated with spontaneous preterm delivery:

86. cocaine abuse throughout pregnancy.
87. placental chorioangioma.
88. placental sulphatase deficiency.

The following statements relating to preterm labour are correct:

89. Beta-sympathomimetic agents used in conjunction with corticosteroids are a recognised cause of maternal pulmonary oedema.
90. Preterm rupture of the membranes is frequently consequent upon orgasm.

The following statements relating to the use of prostaglandins (PG) are correct:

91. PGE_2 0.5 mg vaginally will induce labour in 80% of women with an unripe cervix.
92. $PGF_2\alpha$ is ten times more potent than PGE_2 in inducing contractions.
93. Beta-agonists will suppress the contractions induced by prostaglandins.

The umbilical cord

94. is more likely to prolapse if greater than 35 cm in length.
95. vessels require fetoscopic visualisation prior to cordocentesis.

Early decelerations in the fetal heart rate in labour

96. indicate fetal hypokalaemia.
97. are a sign of fetal hypoxia.

Spinal anaesthesia (subarachnoid block) in obstetric practice

98. is not suitable as an anaesthetic in the manual removal of a retained placenta.

F 99. is associated with less hypotension than is epidural anaesthesia.

Concerning the vaginal delivery of the second twin,

F 100. internal podalic version is no longer an acceptable procedure.

Predisposing factors to face presentation include

T 101. contracted pelvis. ?
T 102. preterm labour.
T 103. fetal goitre.

The following statements regarding occipito-posterior (OP) positions are correct:

T 104. Between 10% and 20% of all cephalic presentations are OP in early labour.
T 105. Less than 10% will deliver spontaneously face-to-pubis.
T 106. Labour is associated with early spontaneous rupture of the membranes.
T 107. In multiparous women, it is the commonest cause of a high head at term. ?

A randomised, double-blind trial was conducted on the use of suture materials X and Y for repairing episiotomies with the addition of an oral anti-inflammatory compound or a placebo. The outcome of the trial was measured by the need for analgesic drugs and the table shows the proportion of women in the four treatment groups who required an analgesic on the second postpartum day.

Treatment Group	Proportion needing Analgesia
a) Suture X + anti-inflammatory drug	27/42 (64.3%)
b) Suture X + placebo	24/42 (57.1%)
	= 51/84 (60.7%)
c) Suture Y + anti-inflammatory drug	22/42 (52.4%)
d) Suture Y + placebo	26/46 (56.5%)
	= 43/53 (54.5%)

The following statements are correct:

F 108. In the comparison of suture X with suture Y, if $P = 0.4$ then the result observed would have occurred by chance on four occasions out of 1000.

F 109. The superiority of suture Y over suture X has been statistically proven.

T 110. Chi-squared is an appropriate statistical test to analyse these data.

In amniotic fluid embolism,

F 111. detection of trophoblastic cells in the peripheral circulation is pathognomonic.

F 112. the patient is likely to be a primigravida.

F 113. over 90% of fatalities occur within one hour of the onset of symptoms.

In the management of massive haemorrhage in the labour ward,

T 114. if additional calcium is needed, then 10% calcium gluconate should be given.

T 115. blood should be administered through blood-warming equipment.

F 116. platelet concentrates should be transfused at an early stage.

Recognised features of massive central pulmonary embolism include

F 117. clinical evidence of deep venous thrombosis in the lower limb in more than 60% of patients.

F 118. pulmonary vascular congestion on the chest X-ray.

T 119. sinus tachycardia.

Acute inversion of the uterus

T 120. occurs most commonly when the placenta is sited in the fundus of the uterus.

Blood loss of more than 500 ml within 12 hours of the delivery of the placenta has a recognised association with

T 121. a low implantation site of the placenta.

T 122. Couvelaire uterus.

T 123. halothane anaesthesia.

F 124. beta-thalassaemia trait.

The following statements referring to mortality statistics, within the UK, are correct:

F 125. Perinatal mortality is defined as the sum of stillbirths and neonatal deaths occurring in the first 28 days of life for each 1000 live births.

T 126. A neonatal death is defined as the death of an infant born alive and who dies within 28 days, irrespective of the stage of gestation.

F 127. A late neonatal death is defined as a death between 14 and 28 days.

T 128. Infant mortality excludes deaths in the first month of life. *(False)*

F 129. A stillbirth is defined as an infant born dead and weighing over 1000 g.

In relation to lactation the following statements are correct:

F 130. Breast engorgement occurs during the first 24 hours following delivery.

When compared with bottle feeding, breastfeeding is associated with a decreased risk of

T 131. sudden infant death syndrome.

T 132. atopic eczema.

The perinatal mortality rate is significantly increased by the following maternal factors:

T 133. chickenpox (varicella) in early pregnancy. *False*

T 134. systemic lupus erythematosus in pregnancy.

The incidence of neonatal respiratory distress syndrome is characteristically increased

F 135. in full-term infants born below the tenth centile for birth weight.

T 136. following prolonged intrauterine hypoxia.

Necrotising enterocolitis is characterised by

T 137. blood in the stool.

T 138. bile-stained vomit.

The following pairs of items are causally linked:

T 139. tracheo-oesophageal fistula : polyhydramnios.

F 140. hypercalcaemia : neonatal convulsions.

T 141. imperforate anus : polyhydramnios.

Recognised associations exist between mid-trimester miscarriage and

F 142. recurrent gonococcal infections.
T 143. bleeding in the first trimester.
T 144. death of one fetus in a twin pregnancy.

Characteristic features of hydatidiform mole include

F 145. bilateral follicular cysts.
F 146. an XY chromosomal karyotype.
T 147. an increased incidence in women over the age of 40 years.

When prostaglandins are used alone for the termination of pregnancy they are associated with

F 148. an induction–abortion interval in the second trimester of under 12 hours in more than 50% of cases.
T 149. hypertension.
F 150. an antidiuretic effect.

The following statements concerning legal termination of pregnancy (in England and Wales) are correct:

F 151. The signatures of two registered medical practitioners, one of whom must be a qualified gynaecologist, are required.
F 152. Rhesus prophylaxis is unnecessary when termination is before eight weeks.

A two-year-old girl has a persistent vaginal discharge that causes vulval irritation and staining of her underwear. The following statements are correct:

T 153. When the discharge is bloodstained, an examination under anaesthesia is required.
F 154. Broad-spectrum antibiotics are the treatment of choice.
T 155. Sexual abuse should be considered as a cause.

Recognised associations of abnormal uterine development include

T 156. acute retention of urine.
T 157. the presence of a pelvic kidney.

Recognised associations of oligomenorrhoea include

T 158. chronic renal failure.
T 159. cystic glandular hyperplasia of the endometrium.

Concerning premature ovarian failure presenting as secondary amenorrhoea in a woman aged 30 years

T 160. less than 10% have a chromosomal aetiology.
T 161. it is clinically indistinguishable from resistant ovarian syndrome.

Uterine fibroids

F 162. are the most common site of leiomyosarcoma development.
F 163. if small and submucous are unlikely to be associated with menorrhagia.
F 164. can be accurately located by pelvic ultrasound.
F 165. if palpable abdominally, should be removed.

Recognised causes of galactorrhoea include

T 166. acromegaly.
T 167. therapy with methyldopa.
T 168. hypothyroidism.

Women with polycystic ovary syndrome are more likely

T 169. if oligomenorrhoeic and obese to achieve a regular cycle by weight reduction alone.
T 170. to have an atherogenic lipid profile than women with normal ovaries.
T 171. to have an elevated plasma testosterone concentration.
T 172. to be hyperinsulinaemic.

A twenty-four-year old woman complains of recent growth of excessive facial and limb hair. Menstruation is normal. Examination confirms the presence of normal breast development, external genitalia and pelvic organs. In relation to this patient, the following statements are correct:

F 173. If all biochemical tests are normal, treatment with cyproterone acetate is indicated.
T 174. Investigation should include pelvic ultrasound.

Obesity is associated with an increased incidence of

T 175. endometrial carcinoma.
F 176. squamous carcinoma of the cervix.

Isolated gonadotrophin deficiency (Kallman syndrome)

F 177. is due to failure of development of the gonadotrophin-producing cells of the pituitary.
F 178. is a recognised cause of secondary amenorrhoea.
T 179. has a recognised association with anosmia.

The following drugs are correctly paired with the side effects indicated:

T 180. mefenamic acid : diarrhoea.
F 181. salazopyrine : impotence.
T 182. oxybutynin hydrochloride : dryness of the mouth.

Acute trichomoniasis in women of reproductive age is characterised by

F 183. a bloodstained vaginal discharge.
F 184. vulval oedema and fissure formation.
F 185. recent ingestion of a broad-spectrum antibiotic.

The following statement regarding genital herpes is correct:

T 186. The acquisition of herpes simplex virus (HSV) type I offers some protection against HSV type II infection.

A 20-year-old married woman presents with a history of offensive irritant vaginal discharge. She has taken a low-dose combined oral contraceptive pill for the last six months. Examination reveals an inflamed cervix and vagina with an offensive discharge. The uterus is anteverted and normal in size but there is general tenderness on pelvic examination. The following statements, relating to this history, are correct:

F 187. A negative high vaginal culture excludes gonococcal infection.
F 188. The signs and symptoms are highly suggestive of cervical ectropion.

The following statements relating to patients with psychosexual problems are correct:

F 189. Successful treatment of vaginismus includes Faradic stimulation of the pelvic floor.

F 190. There is an underlying psychiatric illness in the majority of patients.

If a woman has an increased menstrual flow associated with an intrauterine device, then the following statements are correct:

T 191. Antifibrinolytic agents are of therapeutic value.

F 192. Copper, incorporated into the device, has a haemostatic effect.

The following statements relating to the progestogen-only oral contraceptive are correct:

T 193. Endometrial pseudodecidualisation occurs.

F 194. Lactation is inhibited.

T 195. There is an increase in the incidence of functional ovarian cysts.

In a woman taking a combined oral contraceptive preparation

F 196. there is an increased risk of subarachnoid haemorrhage.

Regarding female laparoscopic tubal occlusion,

F 197. if performed during the luteal phase, uterine curettage reduces the chance of pregnancy.

F 198. if clips were used, failure more than a year later is likely to be the result of misapplication.

T 199. contraception should be continued until the next menstrual period.

The following conditions are correctly paired with an appropriate treatment:

T 200. central (true) precocious puberty : gonadotrophin-releasing hormone analogue.

F 201. premature ovarian failure : clomifene citrate.

Medroxyprogesterone acetate

T 202. is an effective contraceptive agent.

T 203. is associated with breakthrough bleeding.

F 204. induces hypertension.

Gonadotrophin-releasing hormone agonists

F 205. when used in the treatment of endometriosis, require pulsatile administration.

T 206. can be used simultaneously with hormone replacement therapy as appropriate therapy for endometriosis.

A 23-year-old woman, married for three years, complains of primary infertility and amenorrhoea since discontinuing oral contraceptive therapy one year ago. While taking oral contraception her weight increased from 60.8 kg to 74.4 kg (134 lb to 164 lb). Her height is 164 cm (5 feet 6 inches). General systematic and pelvic examinations reveal no abnormality. A diagnostic test for pregnancy carried out on a specimen of urine one week previously was negative. Relevant further investigations include

T 207. serum prolactin estimation.

F 208. serial serum oestradiol estimations.

Concerning the use of clomifene citrate,

F 209. it will induce ovulation in women with anorexia nervosa.

T 210. when used alone it can lead to the development of the ovarian hyperstimulation syndrome.

An initial abnormal seminal analysis requires the following further measures:

F 211. referral for urological investigation.

F 212. the administration of testosterone proprionate.

Concerning in vitro fertilisation,

T 213. the age of the woman influences the pregnancy rate, independent of the number of oocytes recovered.

F 214. oocyte recovery should be attempted within 24 hours of administration of human chorionic gonadotrophin.

F 215. in the UK the replacement of more than three embryos is permitted in exceptional circumstances.

The following statements relating to the menopause are correct:

F 216. Frequency of micturition is a characteristic symptom.
F 217. Atrophic change in the vagina commonly presents with pruritus.
F 218. Obese women are more symptomatic than thin women.

Hormone replacement therapy for the postmenopausal woman is associated with

T 219. a decrease in the concentration of serum follicle-stimulating hormone.
T 220. an increased incidence of coronary artery disease.

Recognised features of pelvic endometriosis include

T 221. an association with low fertility.
T 222. painful defaecation.

Conventional urodynamic studies (dual-channel subtracted cystometry with simultaneous pressure–flow measurements) are essential to distinguish between

F 223. patients with genuine stress incontinence, who would best be treated by surgery, and those where physiotherapy is indicated.
F 224. bacterial cystitis and interstitial cystitis.

Factors which predispose to urinary tract infection include

T 225. renal calculus.

Subsequent genital prolapse may be prevented by

F 226. elective induction of labour at term.
T 227. continuing hormone replacement therapy.

The following statements concerning vulval disorders are correct:

T 228. Paget's disease is associated with apocrine carcinoma.
F 229. Lichen sclerosus should be treated by simple vulvectomy.

An acute tubo-ovarian abscess is associated with

T 230. diarrhoea.
T 231. bacteraemia.
F 232. diagnostic features on ultrasound examination.

149

Regarding the management of a patient after initial treatment for cervical intraepithelial neoplasia,

T 233. the risk of invasive cervical cancer occurring is about five times that of the general population.

T 234. annual smears are recommended for ten years before return to the general screening programme.

F 235. vault smears should be taken for five years after hysterectomy.

Loop diathermy for the management of cervical intraepithelial neoplasia

F 236. utilises a low current to enable an adequate histological interpretation of the excised tissue.

T 237. may be performed at any time during the menstrual cycle.

Carcinoma of the uterine cervix

T 238. characteristically originates from the transformation zone.

F 239. stage II is commonly associated with ureteric obstruction.

F 240. is an adenocarcinoma in less than 10% of cases.

Recognised associations of endometrial hyperplasia include

F 241. prolonged postpartum anovulation.

F 242. Cushing's syndrome.

Endometrial carcinoma

F 243. is histologically well differentiated in the majority of cases.

F 244. has metastasised to the ovaries in approximately 30% of cases at presentation.

F 245. characteristically causes intermenstrual bleeding.

With regard to leiomyosarcoma of the uterus,

T 246. adjuvant pelvic irradiation does not improve survival.

T 247. recurrence of disease occurs in more than 50% of cases.

Benign cystic teratomata (dermoid cysts) of the ovary characteristically

F 248. are associated with menorrhagia.

T 249. have cells containing Barr bodies.

F 250. are multilocular.

T 251. are lined by squamous epithelium.

An ovarian tumour

F 252. when malignant has a significantly improved prognosis if a cytotoxic drug is instilled into the peritoneal cavity at the time of laparotomy.

T 253. undergoes torsion as a recognised complication.

T 254. of the granulosa-cell type causes postmenopausal bleeding.

The following statements concerning epithelial ovarian cancer in the UK are correct:

T 255. Prophylactic bilateral oophorectomy at the time of hysterectomy would prevent about 10% of all cases.

F 256. Second-look laparotomy is justified by an improved five-year survival rate.

F 257. It is associated with prolonged use of a combined oral contraceptive pill.

T 258. It causes more deaths than any other female genital tract cancer.

Regarding prophylaxis against venous thromboembolism in women undergoing gynaecological surgery,

T 259. there is increased risk of wound haematoma if heparin is administered near to the site of an abdominal incision.

T 260. platelet counts should be monitored in patients receiving heparin for more than five days.

T 261. heparin enhances antithrombin III activity.

F 262. dextran 70 acts by activation of coagulation factors.

There is an increased incidence of postoperative 'burst abdomen' in association with

F 263. mass closure techniques.

F 264. non-closure of the parietal peritoneum.

The following statement concerning intestinal obstruction is correct:

F 265. Abdominal distension occurs more often in association with mechanical obstruction than with paralytic ileus.

The following statement relating to abdominal hysterectomy is correct:

T 266. The operation carries less risk to the bowel than does laparoscopy.

Regarding endometrial ablation/resection,

F 267. the risk of fluid overload is avoided by the use of less than five litres of irrigant.

F 268. patients rendered amenorrhoeic following the procedure do not need contraception.

T 269. about 50% of all hysterectomies can be avoided.

T 270. a small proportion of patients will develop cyclical pain.

September 2001

Concerning vaginal ultrasound imaging in early pregnancy,

T 1. absence of cardiac activity in an embryo of 3 cm crown–rump length reliably indicates a nonviable pregnancy.

F 2. cardiac activity will be seen in a viable embryo of 6 mm length. [?]

Concerning ultrasound in pregnancy,

F 3. ultrasound markers may be detected during a second-trimester scan in 70% of fetuses with Down syndrome.

T 4. trisomy 18 is the chromosome abnormality most commonly associated with choroid plexus cysts.

T 5. most fetuses with a nuchal translucency of 2.5 mm or more are normal.

The following conditions can be diagnosed by ultrasound screening of the fetus:

T 6. syndactyly.

F 7. Tay-Sachs disease.

T 8. congenital heart block.

With regard to fetal lumbar meningomyelocele,

F 9. amniocentesis is necessary to make the diagnosis.

The following condition is characteristically associated with oligohydramnios:

T 10. talipes equinovarus.

The following conditions would be expected to conform to the pattern of inheritance shown in Figure 7:

F 11. Huntington's chorea.

T 12. phenylketonuria.

T 13. cystic fibrosis.

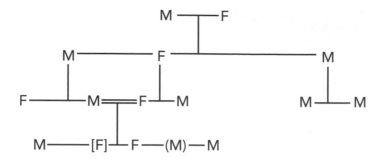

====== : Consanguineous mating

[M = normal male, (M) = affected male, F = normal female, [F] = affected female]

Figure 7

Recognised causes of vomiting in the second trimester of pregnancy include

F   14.   ulcerative colitis.
T   15.   necrobiosis in a fibroid.

The following statements regarding multiple sclerosis in pregnancy are correct:

T   16.   Epidural anaesthesia will not precipitate a relapse.
F   17.   The second stage of labour should be shortened.
T   18.   It has no effect on the long-term prognosis of the disease.

The following have a recognised association:

T   19.   antenatal corticosteroid administration : reduced incidence of neonatal necrotising enterocolitis.
F   20.   donor insemination in natural cycles : increased miscarriage rate.

In maternal thyrotoxicosis complicating pregnancy and the puerperium

F   21.   the condition is best treated by giving a 'blocking' dose of carbimazole together with a normal replacement dose of thyroxine.

F 22. neonatal hyperthyroidism does not occur if the mother has been euthyroid.

T 23. subtotal thyroidectomy is acceptable treatment in the second trimester

The following occurs more frequently in the pregnant than in the nonpregnant woman:

F 24. duodenal ulcer.

Gestational diabetes is characteristically associated with

F 25. a need for treatment with insulin in the majority of cases.

F 26. an increased incidence of neonatal hypercalcaemia.

F 27. an increased incidence of fetal malformation, even when treated.

The following condition has an increased incidence in pregnancy complicated by poorly controlled diabetes mellitus:

T 28. fetal sacral agenesis.

Sickle cell anaemia in pregnant women is associated with an increased incidence of

T 29. intrauterine growth restriction.

T 30. megaloblastic anaemia.

A rhesus negative woman, with rhesus D antibodies, is in the 18th week of her fifth pregnancy. Her last child had haemolytic disease of the newborn and required four postnatal exchange transfusions. This pregnancy is by a different partner whose rhesus genotype is cde/CDE. It therefore follows that.

F 31. a positive indirect Coombs test performed on cord blood indicates a child affected by haemolytic disease.

T 32. if an affected fetus requires an intrauterine transfusion then group O rhesus negative blood should be crossmatched against the mother's serum.

F 33. the infant has a 75% chance of being affected with haemolytic disease.

A healthy normotensive woman aged 40 years is pregnant for the first time. Compared with an otherwise similar 25-year-old woman,

F 34. she is approximately ten times more likely to give birth to a baby with translocation Down syndrome.

T 35. she has almost double the likelihood of a twin pregnancy.
T 36. she has an increased chance of developing a trophoblastic tumour.
F 37. the risk of her baby having a neural tube defect is increased by 10%.

There is a recognised association between intrauterine death of the fetus and

T 38. well-controlled maternal diabetes mellitus.
T 39. external cephalic version.
T 40. infection with *Toxoplasma gondii*.

The following drugs administered during pregnancy are correctly paired with a recognised unwanted side effect:

T 41. carbimazole : fetal goitre.
F 42. 1-thyroxine : neonatal thyrotoxicosis.
F 43. labetalol : meconium ileus.

In the evaluation of abdominal pain at 24 weeks of pregnancy,

F 44. quiescent ulcerative colitis is liable to relapse during pregnancy.
F 45. an ultrasound scan can exclude a placental abruption.
F 46. if appendicitis is suspected, laparoscopy is indicated.

A 30-year-old woman who has had four previous normal pregnancies and deliveries is admitted to hospital at 30 weeks of gestation. For the past four hours she has had severe generalised abdominal pain. On examination she is pale and anxious. Her blood pressure is 110/70 mmHg and her pulse rate is 100 beats per minute. The fundal height is 32 cm above the symphysis pubis. The lie is longitudinal but the presentation is difficult to determine because of marked abdominal tenderness. The fetal heart is not audible and no trace is obtained on cardiotocography. Ultrasound examination confirms fetal death. The haemoglobin is 10 g/dl, the platelet count is 25 x 10⁹/l. Oozing from the site of the venepuncture is noted. The following statements are correct:

F 47. Delivery should be deferred until the platelets and fibrin degradation products concentrations have returned to normal.
F 48. Depletion of factor VIII is likely.
T 49. Urgent transfusion with fresh blood is indicated.
F 50. The most likely diagnosis is ruptured uterus.

The following statements concerning rubella and pregnancy are correct:

F 51. Maternal infection occurring in the second trimester is followed by the neonatal rubella syndrome in less than 1% of cases.

F 52. Treatment with immunoglobulin reduces the risk of congenital abnormality.

F 53. Rubella vaccination is associated with the neonatal rubella syndrome.

Listeria monocytogenes

T 54. multiplies at temperatures as low as six degrees Celsius.

F 55. is spread through droplets in the air.

T 56. is difficult to culture in the laboratory.

The following maternal symptoms have a recognised association with parvovirus B19 infection:

T 57. polyarthropathy.

T 58. transient aplastic anaemia in those with sickle cell anaemia.

Regarding fetal infection with toxoplasmosis,

F 59. the fetus is more severely affected when infection occurs late in pregnancy.

F 60. spiramycin is more effective than pyrimethamine or sulfadiazine in treating the affected fetus.

F 61. pregnancy reactivates latent disease.

Clinical manifestations of neonatal cytomegalovirus infection include

T 62. petechiae.

T 63. cataracts.

The following anti-infective agents are contraindicated in the third trimester of pregnancy:

T 64. chloramphenicol.

F 65. metronidazole.

F 66. acyclovir.

In a paper describing the use of a new drug for the treatment of hypertension in pregnancy you read: 'The mean fall in diastolic blood pressure in the treated group (*n* = 30) was 10 mmHg ± 3.0 (SD) and in a control group given placebo (n = 29) the mean fall was 4 mmHg ± 2.6 (SD). Using the t test, *P* < 0.001'. Assuming a normal distribution, the following statements are correct:

F 67.   The most appropriate way to allocate patients to the drug or the placebo group would have been to give the drug or placebo to alternate patients.

F 68.   If the trial were properly conducted, the doctors involved should know which patients received the active drug and which the placebo.

F 69.   The difference in blood pressure fall fails to reach a significant level.

In the long-term treatment of hypertension in pregnancy

T 70.   hydralazine hydrochloride is an unsuitable drug.

A 23-year-old primigravida with no significant medical history is found to have proteinuria (++) at the booking clinic at 16 weeks. This finding is confirmed on examination of a midstream specimen of urine, which is sterile. Proteinuria persists. The following antenatal investigations are indicated:

T 71.   a 24-hour urine protein estimation.
F 72.   intravenous urography (pyelography).
F 73.   blood clotting screen.

Recognised associations of eclampsia include

T 74.   hypovolaemia.
T 75.   mesenteric arterial thrombosis.

External cephalic version of a singleton breech presentation

F 76.   should only be attempted in conjunction with the use of tocolytic agents.

T 77.   is more likely to be successful in black African than in Caucasian women.

The following conditions have a recognised association with spontaneous preterm labour:

T 78.   fetal oesophageal atresia.

F 79. maternal hypertension.

F 80. teenage pregnancy.

With respect to multiple pregnancy,

T 81. the frequency of monozygotic twins is approximately uniform throughout the world.

F 82. the presence of two separate placentas is diagnostic of dizygotic twins.

When the gestational age is 42 weeks or more

F 83. there is a substantial fall in the fetal haemoglobin concentration.

F 84. the most common cause of perinatal death is trauma.

F 85. there is a significant preponderance of female infants.

Intravaginal prostaglandin E, is significantly associated with

F 86. neonatal hyponatraemia.

F 87. neonatal bronchospasm.

Recognised causes of persistent occipito-posterior position of the fetal head include

F 88. oligohydramnios.

With regard to face presentation at term,

F 89. mento-posterior position is more frequent than mento-anterior position.

F 90. the incidence is increased by the use of epidural analgesia.

F 91. the recorded incidence is approximately 1/150 deliveries.

In labour following one caesarean section,

F 92. the incidence of rupture of a 'classical' scar is approximately 20%.

T 93. fetal heart rate abnormalities indicate the possibility of scar dehiscence.

There is an increased incidence of prolapse of the umbilical cord with

F 94. increasing maternal age.

F 95. circumvallate placenta.

T 96. mento-posterior position. *False*

Fetal acidosis in labour is characteristically associated with

T 97. prolonged uterine hypertonus.

T 98. recurrent late decelerations on a cardiotocographic trace.

The following statements concerning continuous lumbar epidural analgesia are correct:

F 99. The procedure must be abandoned if a spinal tap occurs during its administration.

F 100. It is contraindicated where intrauterine growth restriction is suspected.

T 101. Respiratory arrest is a recognised complication.

F 102. It increases the risk of postpartum haemorrhage.

Acute inversion of the uterus may be associated with active management of the third stage of labour and

T 103. the uterus should be replaced immediately whether or not the placenta has separated.

F 104. is a consequence of waiting overlong for the uterus to contract.

In the management of hypovolaemic shock

F 105. there is negligible risk of acute respiratory distress syndrome (shock lung) unless more than five litres of crystalloid has been transfused.

F 106. there is no danger of pulmonary oedema while the central venous pressure is normal.

T 107. the use of polygeline (Haemaccel) interferes with blood crossmatching.

F 108. the foot of the bed should be raised to improve renal perfusion.

Features of disseminated intravascular coagulation include

F 109. an association with systemic lupus erythematosus.

T 110. activation of factor VII.

T 111. the appearance of free plasmin in the circulation.

Recognised associations of major pulmonary thromboembolism include

F 112. a prolonged clotting time.

T 113. the presence of lupus anticoagulant.

T 114. protein C deficiency.

F 115. early change in the chest X-ray.

According to the international (FIGO) definition, the calculation of the maternal mortality rate

116. excludes deaths due to fortuitous diseases, for example, carcinoma of the stomach.
117. includes only deaths that occur during pregnancy.
118. excludes deaths due to ectopic pregnancy.

Breastfeeding and 'rooming in' (whereby the baby's cot is next to the mother's bed)

119. means the infant is more likely to colonise bacteria from its own mother than from elsewhere.
120. reduces the future incidence of non accidental injury.
121. encourages four-hourly feeding regimens.

Drugs considered to be unsuitable for administration to the breastfeeding mother include

122. rifampicin.
123. senna.
124. combined oral contraceptive pill.
125. pseudoephedrine.

The following statements concerning puerperal mastitis are correct:

126. Suckling should be discouraged on the affected breast.
127. Group A streptococci are the commonest causal organisms.

Perinatal mortality rates (PMR) per 1000 births by birth weight are given for two towns X and Y (actual number of deaths are given in parenthesis). The following statements, which refer to the above data, are correct:

128. A statistical test for differences of PMR is reported as $P > 0.05$. This suggests that by accepted standards the differences are due to chance.
129. It is not possible from the data shown to calculate the overall perinatal mortality rate for town X.
130. Low birth weight ($\leq 2500\,g$) was a factor in one in three perinatal deaths.
131. More babies (live and stillborn) were delivered in town Y than in town X.

The following statements concerning meconium aspiration are correct:

T 132. It can occur prior to labour.
F 133. It is more common following breech delivery.
F 134. It is a common feature of preterm delivery.

Recognised causes of ambiguous genitalia at birth include

F 135. the androgen insensitivity syndrome.
F 136. Klinefelter syndrome.
T 137. severe hypospadias.

Septic termination of pregnancy or miscarriage, when associated with a *Clostridium perfringens* (*welchii*) infection, has the following recognised features:

T 138. jaundice.
T 139. hypotension.
T 140. acute respiratory distress syndrome.

In women with choriocarcinoma

F 141. a rise in the concentration of urinary human chorionic gonadotrophin, after initial clinical response, is diagnostic of recurrence.
F 142. there is usually a recent history of first-trimester miscarriage.

Recognised features of Turner syndrome include.

F 143. a mosaic pattern (45X0/46XX) in approximately 50% of cases.
F 144. absence of withdrawal bleeding after treatment with hormone therapy.

An individual of female phenotype with gonadal dysgenesis and an XY karyotype characteristically

T 145. has a vagina.
F 146. has galactorrhoea.

Regarding precocious puberty,

T 147. it is usually idiopathic.
T 148. failure to treat commonly leads to short stature.
T 149. when idiopathic, it may be treated with cyproterone acetate.

The following statement regarding normal puberty is correct:

F 150. The maximal growth spurt occurs after the menarche.

A 17-year-old girl with no secondary sex characteristics is currently studying for university entrance. She has never menstruated. She is 1.60 m tall, weighs 47.6 kg and has a body mass index of 18.6. Laboratory results are reported as: karyotype XX; plasma follicle-stimulating hormone 5.0 iu/l; plasma luteinising hormone 6.2 iu/l and plasma prolactin 300 mu/l. The following statements are correct:

F 151. The most likely cause of her amenorrhoea is haematocolpos.
F 152. X-ray of the skull is mandatory.
F 153. Laparoscopy is necessary to establish the cause.

Premature ovarian failure

T 154. is a recognised complication of mumps.
F 155. is a characteristic feature of anorexia nervosa.
T 156. does not occur when plasma oestradiol concentrations are normal.

In women with idiopathic heavy menstrual bleeding

T 157. more than 90% are ovulating normally.
F 158. curettage is of therapeutic benefit.

The following symptoms are correctly paired with a recognised cause:

T 159. ptyalism : hyperemesis gravidarum.
F 160. hirsutism : prolactinoma.
F 161. diplopia : avascular necrosis of the pituitary.

The combination of inappropriate lactation and secondary amenorrhoea has a recognised association with

F 162. hyperthyroidism.
T 163. acromegaly.

Recognised associations of polycystic ovary syndrome include

F 164. spasmodic dysmenorrhoea.
F 165. carcinoma of the breast.

Prolactin secretion is inhibited by

F 166. lithium carbonate.
T 167. cabergoline.
T 168. quinagolide.

An 18-year-old woman presents with right iliac fossa pain and a heavy vaginal discharge. Her last menstrual period was six weeks earlier. She had been regularly taking a combined oral contraceptive for the past eight months. She is apyrexial. Abdominal examination reveals a poorly localised area of tenderness in the right iliac fossa. Vaginal examination shows no abnormality. Results of investigation include: urine microscopy – numerous pus cells, haemoglobin 9 g/dl, white cell count 8.4 x 10⁹/l. The following courses of action are appropriate:

F 169. Perform a plain X-ray of the abdomen.
F 170. Arrange urgent laparoscopy.
F 171. Prescribe antibiotics.

The incidence of vaginal candidiasis is increased

F 172. in postmenopausal women.
F 173. in women who wear dentures.

Procedures of value in the diagnosis of gonorrhoea in the female include

F 174. culture of a high vaginal swab.
F 175. naked-eye examination of the vaginal discharge.

Bacterial vaginosis

T 176. is unlikely with a vaginal pH below 4.5.
T 177. is associated with an increased number of anaerobes.
T 178. can be successfully treated with intravaginal clindamycin.

The following statements concerning the human immunodeficiency virus are correct:

F 179. Sexual transmission is reduced by the use of spermicides.
T 180. The spread of infection to healthcare attendants is lessened by the measures which are effective against the spread of hepatitis B.

Contraindications to the use of an intrauterine contraceptive device include

F 181. herpes simplex (type II) infection.
F 182. continuous salicylate therapy.

Following the insertion of an intrauterine contraceptive device

F 183. the expulsion rate during the first year is at least 20%.
F 184. a typical pregnancy rate during the first year is 4/100 women years.

The following metabolic changes occur with the use of the combined oral contraceptive pill:

F 185. angiotensin II activity falls.
T 186. endogenous progesterone concentrations fall.
T 187. serum ferritin concentrations rise.

The following statements about methods of contraception are correct:

T 188. Oil-based creams and gels adversely affect the efficacy of the male condom.
F 189. Most diaphragms are impregnated with nonoxynol-9.

With laparoscopic clip sterilisation

F 190. the procedure should not be performed during menstruation.
F 191. there is less morbidity than with vasectomy.

The following conditions are correctly paired with a recognised cause:

T 192. reversible oligozoospermia : sulfasalazine.
T 193. asthenospermia : Kartagener syndrome.
T 194. impotence : hyperprolactinaemia.

Clomifene citrate is a recognised treatment for

F 195. oligozoospermia associated with a raised serum follicle-stimulating hormone concentration.
F 196. galactorrhoea.
F 197. adenomyosis.

Assisted conception using ovum donation should be considered in women with

F 198. Asherman syndrome.
F 199. androgen insensitivity.
F 200. congenital uterine anomalies.

With regard to endometriosis,

F 201. its incidence is increased following prenatal exposure to diethylstilboestrol.
T 202. medroxyprogesterone acetate is a recommended drug in the treatment of symptomatic mild to moderate disease.
T 203. it is more common in women with müllerian duct abnormalities.

Recognised complications of pelvic endometriosis include

F 204. vaginal adenosis.
F 205. postmenopausal bleeding.
T 206. hydronephrosis.

Recognised side effects of the administration of danazol include

F 207. weight loss.
T 208. dryness of the vagina.
F 209. galactorrhoea.

Gonadotrophin-releasing hormone analogue administration

F 210. should be discontinued if ovarian hyperstimulation occurs.
F 211. is associated with an increased incidence of acne vulgaris.
F 212. within two weeks of conception will result in miscarriage.

Recognised causes of postmenopausal bleeding include

F 213. preinvasive carcinoma of the cervix.
F 214. benign teratoma of the ovary.
F 215. subserous fibroids.
T 216. hepatic cirrhosis.

A 60-year-old married woman presents with a history of recent vaginal bleeding. On examination, the cervix appears healthy, the uterus is small and atrophic and no abnormality is felt in the adnexa. A cervical smear is reported as showing cells suspicious of malignancy, possibly columnar. In the management of this patient

F 217. the smear should be repeated prior to further investigation.

F 218. cone biopsy is appropriate treatment.

F 219. adenocarcinoma of the endocervix is the most likely diagnosis.

A postmenopausal woman exhibits the following change:

T 220. atrophic trigonitis of the bladder.

Oestrogen replacement therapy is of value in

F 221. lichen sclerosus et atrophicus.

F 222. alopecia areata.

Frequency of micturition is a recognised feature of

T 223. papilloma of the bladder.

F 224. vesicovaginal fistula.

Urodynamic studies

F 225. can distinguish between neuropathic and idiopathic detrusor instability.

F 226. reveal that genuine stress incontinence only occurs when the intravesical pressure is in excess of 30 cm water.

F 227. necessitate the use of video equipment.

The aims of surgery for the relief of stress incontinence of urine include

F 228. reduction of the functional length of the urethra.

T 229. an increase in urethral resistance.

The following may lead to genital prolapse in parous women:

T 230. pudendal nerve damage.

Genital prolapse is best treated non-surgically

F 231. in a patient with recurrent prolapse after vaginal hysterectomy and repair .

The following are correctly paired:

T 232. recurrent ulceration of the labia minora : Behcet's disease.

The vulval skin

F 233. contains cellular atypia in more than 25% of cases of lichen sclerosus et atrophicus.

F 234. when affected by lichen sclerosus et atrophicus responds to local testosterone preparations.

T 235. is a site for psoriasis.

In primary carcinoma of the fallopian tube

F 236. the tumour is bilateral in approximately 60% of cases. *(False - 20%)*

F 237. transcoelomic spread rarely occurs.

F 238. radiotherapy is the treatment of choice.

T 239. a profuse watery vaginal discharge is a characteristic symptom.

Cervical ectopy

F 240. is more common in progestogen-only oral contraceptive users than in users of intrauterine contraceptive devices.

F 241. has the histological features of an ulcer.

A 25-year-old parous woman whose cervical smear showed moderate and then severe dyskaryosis has a colposcopic examination that shows no abnormality. The following treatments are appropriate:

F 242. knife conisation.

F 243. a repeat smear in three months' time.

F 244. laser vaporisation.

A 45-year-old woman is found to have a friable tumour on the anterior lip of the cervix with extension to the left parametrium. Histology of the tumour is squamous-cell carcinoma. An intravenous urogram shows a left hydroureter and left hydronephrosis. Cystoscopy reveals bullous oedema. The following statements are correct:

F 245. A diagnosis of stage IV carcinoma of the cervix can be made with confidence.

T 246. The patient's blood urea is likely to be normal.

In stage IIb carcinoma of the cervix

T 247. radiotherapy is the treatment of choice.

F 248. colposcopy is indicated before treatment.

With regard to adenocarcinoma of the uterus,

F 249. the removal of a vaginal cuff at the time of hysterectomy for stage I disease reduces the incidence of vault recurrence.

F 250. preoperative treatment with progestogens improves the prognosis.

F 251. uterine size is a reliable prognostic indicator.

Endometrial carcinoma

F 252. metastasises characteristically to the supraclavicular lymph nodes.

F 253. is a sequel to prenatal oestrogen therapy.

With regard to serum tumour markers in ovarian malignancy,

F 254. a raised serum CA125 concentration is found in association with approximately 40% of epithelial tumours.

F 255. carcino-embryonic antigen (CEA) concentration is more commonly raised in association with serous than with mucinous tumours.

T 256. CA125 concentration is a less specific marker before the menopause.

Five-year survival in stage III ovarian cancer is improved by

F 257. adjuvant pelvic radiotherapy.

F 258. para-aortic lymphadenectomy.

F 259. intraperitoneal alkylating agents.

The following have a recognised association:

F 260. ulcerative colitis : radiological 'skip lesions'.
T 261. diverticular disease : vaginal fistula formation.
F 262. colorectal carcinoma : vegetarianism.

Cryosurgery is recognised as effective in the treatment of

F 263. vulval intraepithelial neoplasia (VIN).
F 264. cervical intraepithelial neoplasia stage 3 (CIN3).

For the first 18 hours after a difficult abdominal hysterectomy a patient fails to void urine. The following statements are correct:

F 265. The most likely cause is prolonged hypovolaemia.
T 266. If due to ureteric injury, she should be treated by nephrostomies and definitive ureteric repair three months later.
F 267. She is best managed by dialysis until the diagnosis is established.

The following are recognised causes of a delay of more than 30 minutes in the recovery after genera anaesthesia:

T 268. severe hypoxia during anaesthesia.
F 269. perioperative blood transfusion of more than three units.
T 270. concurrent use of hypotensive drugs.

Index

abdominal pain
  acute 102
  bilateral lower 98
  in pregnancy 48, 68–9, 136, 156
  vaginal discharge with 76–7, 164
abscess
  pelvic 27, 115
  tubo-ovarian 62, 149
achondroplasia 1, 85
acidosis, fetal intrapartum 72, 160
adenocarcinoma
  cervix 13, 100
  ovary 101
  uterus 81–2, 169
adolescent girls
  imperforate vagina 43, 130
  pelvic mass 41, 129
  short stature 25
  see also girls, young
adrenal carcinoma 46, 134
adrenal hyperplasia, congenital 112, 134
adrenal tumours 31
adriamycin 100
age, maternal see maternal age
alphafetoprotein, serum 7, 101
ambiguous genitalia 74, 162
amenorrhoea
  post-pill 60, 148
  primary 13, 75, 94, 163
  secondary see secondary
    amenorrhoea
  weight-related 9
amniocentesis 33, 121
  diagnostic 1, 19–20, 103
amniotic fluid
  analysis 1, 84, 103
  embolism 54, 90, 122, 142
  infection 7, 20
anaemia
  megaloblastic 17
  in pregnancy 17, 107
anaesthesia, delayed recovery 83, 170
androgen insensitivity syndrome 11,

39–40, 46, 127
  complete 111, 134
anencephaly 37, 125
anorexia nervosa 46, 134
anosmia 9
anovulation 9
antenatal screening test 3, 39, 127
anticoagulation 17, 88
anti-D immunoglobulin 4
antidiuretic hormone, inappropriate
    secretion 46, 112, 134
anti-infective agents, in pregnancy 70,
    157
anus, imperforate 56, 143
aspiration of gastric contents, during
    labour 2, 91
assisted conception 78, 114, 166
asthenospermia 78, 165
athletes, female 112
autosomal recessive diseases 1–2, 35,
    105, 123
azoospermia 14, 41, 114, 129

bacterial vaginosis 27, 77, 96, 164
bacteriuria, asymptomatic 34, 106, 122
beta-agonists (betamimetics) 35, 108, 123
    see also ritodrine
beta-haemolytic streptococcus 4
birth weight 3
borderline epithelial tumours of ovary 24
bottle feeding 55, 143
breast carcinoma 101
breast cysts 31, 118
breastfeeding 91–2
    benefits 55, 73, 143, 161
    drugs during 6, 38, 73, 110, 126, 161
    see also lactation
breast milk 6, 110
breech presentation 5, 70–1, 91, 158
'burst' abdomen, postoperative 64, 151

CA125, serum 24, 117
caesarean section 90

previous 7, 72, 109, 159
cancers, female 25, 118
candidiasis, vaginal 77, 164
cardiac arrest 102
cardiomyopathy, peripartum 51, 138–9
cardiovascular disease, and pregnancy 107
cardiovascular system, in pregnancy 22
cerebral palsy 3
cervical canal, sperm transport 42, 129
cervical carcinoma 31, 62, 100, 150
    adenocarcinoma 13, 100
    advanced 81, 169
    pelvic irradiation 24
        radiotherapy vs radical hysterectomy 27
    stage IIb 11, 169
cervical cerclage, abdominal 19
cervical ectopy (erosion) 15, 81, 168
cervical intraepithelial neoplasia (CIN) 23, 62, 100, 117, 150
cervical smears
    abnormal 117
    borderline 117
    dyskaryosis 81, 168
    identifiable infections 46, 133
    suspicious cells 79, 167
chemotherapy 28, 31
children see girls, young
chlamydial infection 27, 115
cholestasis, intrahepatic, of pregnancy 2, 22, 86, 106
chorioadenoma destruens 114
chorioamnionitis 20, 89
chorioangioma, placental 51, 90
choriocarcinoma 24, 75, 94, 114, 134, 162
chorionic villus sampling (CVS) 19, 84
cisplatin(um) 45, 133
climacteric 14, 98
clinical trials 21–2, 54, 70, 89–90, 141–2, 158
clomifene citrate 14, 60, 78, 114–15, 148, 165
Clostridium perfringens (welchii) infection 13, 74, 162
coeliac disease 50
colorectal carcinoma 82, 170
colposcopy 81, 117
condylomata accuminata 15
cone biopsy 100
Confidential Enquiries into Maternal Deaths 110
congenital adrenal hyperplasia 112, 134
congenital dislocation of hip 18, 110

contraception 13, 78, 165
corticosteroids (glucocorticoids), antenatal 37, 48, 125, 136, 154
Crohn's disease 34–5, 82
cryosurgery 82, 170
curettage, uterine 44, 132
cystocele 98
cystometry, dual-channel 14
    see also urodynamic studies
cytomegalovirus (CMV)
    congenital 33, 86, 121
    infection in pregnancy 49, 137
    neonatal infection 69, 157
cytotoxic therapy 101

danazol 79, 95, 111, 166
deep vein thrombosis 86, 119
dermoid cysts, ovarian 30, 63, 150
detrusor instability 116
diabetes mellitus
    gestational 67, 87, 155
    insulin-dependent
        pregnancy in 51, 67, 88, 107, 139, 155
        secondary amenorrhoea 40–1, 128
diethylstilboestrol 28, 99
diplopia 9, 76, 163
disseminated intravascular coagulation 4, 33, 73, 109, 121, 160
diverticular disease 82, 170
donor insemination 154
Down syndrome 47, 85, 135
    clinical features 35, 123
    risk assessment 38, 126
    translocation 18, 105
doxorubicin hydrochloride 100
drugs
    breastfeeding mothers 6, 38, 73, 110, 126, 161
    inhibiting prolactin secretion 76, 164
    placental transfer 32–3, 108, 120–1
    side effects 58, 68, 95, 146, 156
    in third trimester 52, 70, 140
Duchenne muscular dystrophy 38, 104, 125
ductus arteriosus, persistent 18, 92
duodenal ulcer 67, 155
dysgerminomas, ovarian 12, 101
dysmenorrhoea
    primary 43–4, 113, 131
    secondary 14, 95
dyspareunia 98

eclampsia 22, 90
    associations 51, 70, 158
    drug treatment 50, 138
ectopic pregnancy 93, 114
Eisenmenger syndrome 138
ejaculation, retrograde 96
elderly primigravida 8, 68, 155–6
endometrial ablation/resection 64, 152
endometrial carcinoma 63, 82, 101, 150, 169
    extrapelvic recurrence 117
    metastases 12
    risk factors 10, 24, 44, 100, 117, 131
    stage and spread 31
endometrial hyperplasia 44, 63, 131, 150
    atypical 12, 100
endometriosis 78–9, 98, 166
    pelvic 61, 149, 166
enterocele 43, 98, 115, 130
epidural analgesia 21, 66, 72, 91, 110, 160
epilepsy, maternal 17, 51, 139
erectile impotence 29, 78, 165
ergometrine, intravenous 5
erythema nodosum 67
external cephalic version 4, 52, 70–1, 92, 109, 139, 158
eye damage, fetal 5, 105

face presentation 53, 71, 141, 159
fallopian tube 116–17
    infections 30
    primary carcinoma 9, 81, 99, 168
female sterilisation 60, 78, 97, 147, 165
fetal abnormalities/malformations
    antenatal diagnosis 65, 84, 103, 122, 153
    risk factors 6, 36, 48, 124, 136
fetal acidosis, intrapartum 72, 160
fetal alcohol syndrome 48, 136
fetal blood sampling, antenatal 84, 104
fetal growth 3
    see also intrauterine growth restriction
fetal heart 37, 103, 125
fetal heart rate, early decelerations in labour 53, 140
fibroids, uterine 46, 48, 57, 134, 136, 145
folic acid supplements 20, 88, 108
follicle-stimulating hormone (FSH), serum 14, 25, 41, 112, 114, 129
forceps delivery 4, 33, 121
frequency of micturition 80, 99, 167

galactorrhoea 41, 57, 128, 145

gastrointestinal disorders, vulval involvement 26
gastroschisis 7
general anaesthesia, delayed recovery 83, 170
genetic disorders see inheritance
genital herpes 59, 146
genitalia, ambiguous 74, 162
genital prolapse 62, 80, 167–8
genuine stress incontinence 15, 43, 99, 116, 130
gestational age
    42 weeks 71, 159
    uncertain 47, 135
gestational diabetes 67, 87, 155
girls, young
    vaginal bleeding 25, 94
    vaginal discharge 57, 94, 111, 144
    see also adolescent girls
glucocorticoids see corticosteroids
glucose tolerance, impaired 67
gonadal dysgenesis
    pure 46, 134
    XY 75, 162
gonadotrophin-releasing hormone (GnRH)
    agonists/analogues 60, 79, 95–6, 148, 166
gonadotrophins
    isolated deficiency 9, 46, 58, 134, 146
    raised serum levels 95
    see also follicle-stimulating hormone; human chorionic gonadotrophin; luteinising hormone
gonorrhoea 42, 77, 130, 164
Gram-negative septicaemia 97
granulomatous lesions, vulva 26
granulosa-cell ovarian tumours 118
group B streptococcus 106
gynaecological surgery
    postoperative 'burst' abdomen 64, 151
    venous thromboembolism prophylaxis 64, 151

haematuria, painless 13
haemolytic disease of newborn 36, 123
    rhesus see rhesus haemolytic disease
haemorrhage, massive obstetric 20, 54, 142
heart, fetal see fetal heart
herpes, genital 59, 146
hip, congenital dislocation 18, 110
hirsutism, female 95
    adrenal tumours causing 31

associations 76, 112, 163
idiopathic 15, 46
management 58, 145
primary amenorrhoea with 94
Hodgkin's disease 39, 126
hormone replacement therapy (HRT) 61, 98, 149
continuous combined 23
risks and benefits 28
therapeutic value 80, 167
human chorionic gonadotrophin (hCG), serum 20, 103
human immunodeficiency virus (HIV) 27, 49–50, 77, 96–7, 137, 164
hydatidiform mole 56, 114, 144
complete 15, 44, 93–4, 131
hydrocephalus 37, 125
hydrops fetalis, non-immune 19, 38, 47, 92, 110, 135
21-hydroxylase deficiency 112, 134
hypercalcaemia 56, 143
hyperemesis gravidarum 19
hyperprolactinaemia 25, 112
hypertension, pregnancy-induced see pregnancy-induced hypertension
hyperthyroidism (thyrotoxicosis), maternal associations 39, 86, 126
management 16, 67, 87, 154–5
hypovolaemic shock 72, 160
hysterectomy
abdominal 64, 82, 119, 151, 170
radical, in cervical carcinoma 27
vaginal 98, 102
hysteroscopy, diagnostic 118

ileus, postoperative paralytic 102
iliac fossa pain, right 48, 76–7, 136, 164
immunotherapy, recurrent miscarriage 4, 92
impotence, erectile 29, 78, 165
incision, transverse suprapubic 102
incontinence, urinary
dribbling 99
stress see stress incontinence
urge 12
induction of labour 52, 92, 108, 140
infant mortality 55, 143
infections
amniotic fluid 7, 20
fetal, eye damage 5, 105
maternal, in pregnancy 8, 36, 49, 124, 137
see also specific infections
infertility 11, 42, 60

male 14, 29, 41–2, 61, 96, 114
post-pill 11, 60, 113, 148
see also amenorrhoea
inflammatory bowel disease 34–5, 106
inheritance 48, 136
autosomal recessive 1–2, 35, 105, 123
modes 37, 47, 85, 124, 135
patterns 6–7, 36, 66, 85, 104, 124, 153–4
X-linked 16, 105
intermenstrual bleeding 76
intestinal obstruction 10, 64, 119, 151
intracytoplasmic sperm injection (ICSI) 114
intrahepatic cholestasis of pregnancy 2, 22, 86, 106
intrauterine contraceptive device (IUCD) 97, 113, 165
complications 10
contraindications 77
increased menstrual flow 59, 147
management 30
intrauterine death 68, 156
intrauterine growth restriction 47, 84, 135
intrauterine insemination 29, 96
intravenous infusion, prolonged maternal 66
in vitro fertilisation 61, 96, 148

jaundice, neonatal 1, 4, 19, 92–3, 111

Kallman syndrome (isolated gonadotrophin deficiency) 9, 46, 58, 134, 146
Kielland forceps delivery 33, 121
Klinefelter syndrome 46, 94, 134
Krukenberg tumours 45, 132

labia minora, recurrent ulceration 80, 168
labour
aspiration of gastric contents 2, 91
fetal acidosis 72, 160
induction 52, 92, 108, 140
intramuscular pethidine 22, 89
preterm see preterm labour
prolonged first stage 91
third stage management 5, 72, 91, 160
lactation 55, 143
inappropriate 41, 76, 129, 163
see also breastfeeding; galactorrhoea
laparoscopy
clip sterilisation 78, 165
complications 10

tubal occlusion 147
leiomyosarcoma, uterine 63, 150
lichen sclerosus, vulval 26
Listeria (monocytogenes) infection 17, 69, 86, 106, 157
loop diathermy 62, 150
lupus erythematosus, systemic 34, 86, 87
luteinising hormone (LH), serum 12, 29, 112

male infertility 14, 29, 41–2, 61, 96, 114
mastitis, puerperal 8, 73, 161
maternal age
    38 years 47, 135
    40 years 8, 68, 155–6
    over 35 years 4, 21, 35, 89, 108, 123
maternal deaths 110
maternal mortality rate 73, 161
meconium aspiration 74, 162
medroxyprogesterone acetate 60, 147
megaloblastic anaemia 17
meningomyelocele, fetal lumbar 65, 153
menopause 61, 149
    premature 39, 127
    see also ovarian failure
menstrual bleeding, heavy 97, 115
    idiopathic 44, 76, 132, 163
    IUCD user 59, 147
menstrual irregularities
    athletes 112
    post-pill 11, 113
migraine 66
miscarriage 93
    first trimester 93
    mid-trimester 56, 144
    recurrent 4, 92
    septic 74, 162
mitral stenosis 39, 126
monozygotic twinning 20, 108
monozygotic twin pregnancy 51, 139
mortality statistics 55, 142–3
multiple pregnancy 71, 159
    see also twin pregnancy
multiple sclerosis 66, 154
muscular dystrophy, Duchenne 38, 104, 125
myomectomy 97
myotonic dystrophy 107

necrotising enterocolitis 7, 56, 143
neonatal death 55, 143
neonatal jaundice 1, 4, 19, 92–3, 111
neonate
    ambiguous genitalia 74, 162

'rooming in' 73, 161
neurofibromatosis 50, 138
nuchal translucency 3, 84

obesity 58, 146
oblique lie 21, 109–10
occipitoposterior (OP) positions 53, 71, 141, 159
oestrogen
    replacement therapy *see* hormone replacement therapy
    secreting ovarian tumours 45, 132
older women, pregnancy in *see under* maternal age
oligohydramnios 65, 153
oligomenorrhoea 57, 145
oligozoospermia 42, 78, 96, 129, 165
oocyte retrieval 29
oophorectomy, bilateral 45, 132
oral contraceptive pill
    combined 59, 78, 147, 165
    infertility after discontinuation 11, 60, 113, 148
    progestogen-only 30, 42, 59, 113, 129, 147
osteoporosis 14
ovarian cancer 101
    adenocarcinoma 101
    associations 46, 134
    epithelial 63, 151
    FIGO classification 44, 132
    serum tumour markers 82, 169
    stage III 82, 169
    treatment 24, 101, 118
ovarian dermoid cysts (cystic teratomata) 30, 63, 150
ovarian failure
    premature *see* premature ovarian failure
    primary 8, 60
    secondary 8
    see also menopause
ovarian hyperstimulation syndrome 96
ovarian tumours 63, 101, 132–3, 151
    under 20 years of age 45, 132
    borderline epithelial 24
    dysgerminomas 12, 101
    granulosa-cell 118
    Krukenberg 45, 132
    oestrogen secreting 45, 132
    thecomas 45, 133
    see also ovarian cancer
ovulation stimulation 96
ovum donation 78, 166

oxytocin, intravenous infusion 33, 91, 108, 121

parvovirus (B19) infection 69, 157
patent ductus arteriosus, persistent 18, 92
paternity 48, 136
pelvic abscess 27, 115
pelvic mass, adolescent girl 41, 129
pelvic surgery, complications 26–7
pelvis, bony 32, 120
peptic ulceration 138
perinatal mortality 8, 55, 110, 142
perinatal mortality rate 74, 143
petechiae, vaginal 80
pethidine, intramuscular 22, 89
phaeochromocytoma 33, 106, 121
phenytoin 1
phototherapy 92
pituitary prolactinoma 25
placental abruption 22, 49, 89, 136–7
placental chorioangioma 51, 90
placental transfer 32–3, 108, 120–1
polycystic ovary syndrome 28, 58, 145
    associations 46, 76, 134, 163
polyhydramnios 20, 32, 89, 120
postcoital bleeding 30
postmenopausal bleeding 10, 29, 79, 115, 166–7
postmenopausal women 79, 115, 167
    see also hormone replacement therapy
postpartum haemorrhage 55, 90, 142
post-term pregnancy 71, 159
precocious puberty 8, 40, 75, 128, 162
    central 60, 147
pre-eclampsia 6, 34, 109, 122
pregnancy-induced hypertension
    associations 2
    drug therapy 50, 70, 138, 158
    proteinuric see pre-eclampsia
prelabour rupture of membranes 7
premature ovarian failure 39, 76, 127, 147, 163
    diagnosis 30
    woman aged 30 years 57, 145
preterm baby 19, 36, 93, 111, 123
preterm delivery 52, 140
    breech presentation 91
    forceps 4
preterm labour 2, 120
    inhibition see beta-agonists
    predisposing factors 32, 52, 71, 109, 140, 158–9

progestogen-only contraceptive pill 30, 42, 59, 113, 129, 147
prolactin
    secretion inhibitors 76, 164
    serum 11, 95
prolactinoma, pituitary 25
prolapse
    genital 62, 80, 149, 167–8
    umbilical cord 72, 159
    urethral mucosal 98
prolonged pregnancy 71, 159
prostaglandin E_1 159
prostaglandin E_2 71, 108
prostaglandins 52, 56, 140, 144
proteinuria 6, 34, 70, 109, 158
pruritus ani 14, 99
pruritus vulvae 99, 116
pseudomyxoma peritonei 31, 118
psychosexual problems 59, 147
ptyalism 163
puberty
    delayed female 26, 75
    normal 75, 163
    precocious see precocious puberty
pulmonary embolism, massive central 54, 142
pulmonary oedema 88
pulmonary thromboembolism
    associations 18, 73, 160
    during pregnancy 34, 106, 122
pyelonephritis, acute 34, 87, 122
pyometra 43, 131
pyuria 99

radiotherapy, cervical carcinoma 24, 27
randomised controlled trials 21–2, 54, 89–90, 141–2
respiratory distress syndrome, neonatal 37, 56, 125, 143
retroperitoneal sarcoma 46
rhesus haemolytic disease 6, 18, 67–8, 111, 155
rhesus incompatibility 49, 137
rhesus prophylaxis 4
ritodrine 2, 23, 88
    see also beta-agonists
'rooming in' 73, 161
rubella
    congenital 4–5, 35, 105, 122
    infection in first trimester 2–3, 50, 138
    and pregnancy 69, 157
rupture of membranes, prelabour 7

sacral agenesis 37, 125, 155

salpingitis 28, 97
sarcoidosis 50, 138
screening test, antenatal 3, 39, 127
secondary amenorrhoea 40–1, 128
    after chemotherapy 28
    associations 13, 95, 127
    inappropriate lactation and 76, 129, 163
    premature ovarian failure 57, 145
seminal analysis 61, 148
septic abortion/miscarriage 13, 74, 162
septicaemia, Gram-negative 97
sexual dysfunction 42, 96, 130
shock, hypovolaemic 72, 160
short stature 25
shoulder dystocia 90, 123
sickle cell disease, maternal 50, 138, 139
    complications 18, 51, 67, 87, 139, 155
sickle cell haemoglobin C disease 4, 107
smoking, cigarette 88
sperm transport 42, 129
spinal analgesia/anaesthesia 53, 140–1
statistical analysis 21–2, 54, 70, 74, 89–90, 141–2, 158, 161
sterilisation, female 60, 78, 97, 147, 165
stilboestrol 94
stillbirth 55, 143
streptococcus
    beta-haemolytic 4
    group B 106
stress incontinence 80, 167
    genuine see genuine stress incontinence
subarachnoid block 53, 140–1
suture materials 27
systemic lupus erythematosus 34, 86, 87

teratomata, ovarian cystic 30, 63, 150
termination of pregnancy 56, 113–14, 144
    blood loss 93
    septic 162
testicular feminisation syndrome see androgen insensitivity syndrome
thalassaemia major 87
thecomas, ovarian 45, 133
thrombocytopenic purpura, idiopathic 139
thromboembolism see pulmonary thromboembolism; venous thromboembolism
thyrotoxicosis see hyperthyroidism
tocolytic agents 88
    see also beta-agonists; ritodrine
toxic shock syndrome 42, 130

toxoplasmosis 17
    congenital 86
    fetal infection 69, 157
    and pregnancy 5, 8, 49, 105, 137
tracheo-oesophageal fistula 56, 143
transcervical resection of endometrium 118
transverse lie 32, 91, 120
transverse suprapubic incision 102
trichomoniasis 58, 146
triple X karyotype 23, 94
trophoblastic disease 43, 131
tubal pregnancy 93, 114
tuberculosis, female genital 12, 115
tubo-ovarian abscess 62, 149
tumour markers, serum 82, 169
Turner syndrome
    antenatal diagnosis 84
    features 11, 75, 111, 162
    management 40, 128
twinning, monozygotic 20, 108
twin pregnancy
    monozygotic 51, 139
    vaginal delivery 53, 126, 141
    see also multiple pregnancy

ulcerative colitis 34–5, 106, 170
ultrasound
    antenatal 65, 84, 103, 122, 153
    vaginal see vaginal ultrasound
umbilical arterial Doppler 92
umbilical cord 52, 140
    prolapse 72, 159
ureter, surgical injury 26–7, 170
ureterovaginal fistula 26
urethral mucosal prolapse 98
urge incontinence 12
urinary incontinence see incontinence, urinary
urinary tract infections 62, 149
urobilinogen, urinary 34
urodynamic studies 61, 80, 116, 149, 167
uterine bleeding see vaginal bleeding
uterine curettage 44, 132
uteroplacental blood flow 5, 89, 109
uterus
    abnormal development 57, 144
    acute inversion 6, 55, 72, 142, 160
    adenocarcinoma 81–2, 169
    fibroids see fibroids, uterine
    leiomyosarcoma 63, 150
    ruptured 69, 156

vaccination 16, 86

vacuum extraction 33, 121
vagina
    imperforate 43, 130
    petechiae 80
vaginal adenosis 23
vaginal bleeding
    intermenstrual 76
    irregular, woman aged 45 years 98
    postcoital 30
    postmenopausal see postmenopausal
        bleeding
    young girl 25, 94
vaginal carcinoma 23
vaginal delivery
    transmission of maternal infections 8,
        49, 137
    twins 53, 126, 141
vaginal discharge
    2-year old girl 57, 111, 144
    abdominal pain with 76–7, 164
    offensive irritant 59, 146
    post hysterectomy 119
    pre-menarche 94
vaginal intraepithelial neoplasia (VAIN)
    116
vaginal ultrasound 15, 65
    in early pregnancy 65, 153
vasectomy 9, 113

venous thromboembolism
    postoperative 28
    prophylaxis 64, 151
    see also pulmonary thromboembolism
venous thrombosis, deep 86, 119
vomiting, second trimester 66, 154
von Willebrand's disease 50
vulva
    disorders 62, 149
    gastrointestinal conditions affecting
        26
    granulomatous lesions 26
    lichen sclerosus 26
    malignant disease 99, 116
    noncystic lesions 46, 133
    skin disorders 80–1, 168
    ulceration 46, 133
vulvovaginitis 80

warfarin 17, 88
weight loss 40–1, 128
weight-related amenorrhoea 9
wound healing 27

X-linked disorders 16, 105
XXX karyotype 23, 94
XY gonadal dysgenesis 75, 162